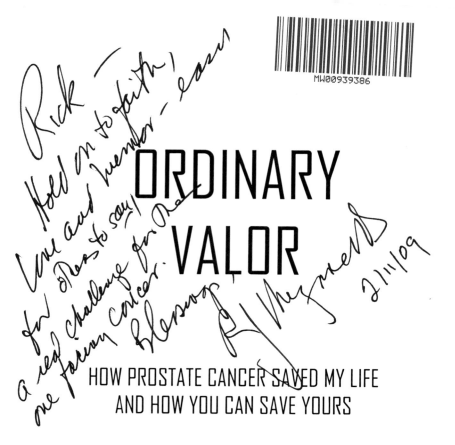

ORDINARY VALOR

HOW PROSTATE CANCER SAVED MY LIFE AND HOW YOU CAN SAVE YOURS

ROBERT J. MIGNONE, M.D., F.A.P.A.

Outskirts Press, Inc.
Denver, Colorado

Outskirts Press
http://www.outskirtspress.com

ISBN-13: 978-1-59800-930-9

Table of Contents

PREFACE i

INTRODUCTION v

PART ONE: BOOM

CHAPTER ONE 1
The Biopsy Result

I barely heard the sound as the concussive wave knocked me back on my heels and stunned all my faculties. The Grim Reaper loomed amongst the swirling shards and debris. My God, is this it?

PART TWO: COLLECTING MYSELF

CHAPTER TWO 19
Walking the Beach

I must regroup fast: gather my wits, clear the smoke, and see myself clearly. I can't afford more "Superdoc" nonsense. Dare to reach out for Susan. And deal with The Boss.

CHAPTER THREE 31
The Ride Home

On my way to tell Susan, I lost myself in reverie about what may be the last delicious memories of our happy homes. Next might come nursing homes.

CHAPTER FOUR......................................39
Breaking the News to Susan

Trembling and sweating, I eked out the "C" word. She pulled me to her breast. Then she cracked me up. Guffaws and tears, doubts and promises. The first big hurdle was cleared.

CHAPTER FIVE 49
Telling the Children

Marcus, Paul, Polly, and Zak. Don't just inform; ask to be loved. Easier said than done.

CHAPTER SIX......................................57
Connecting with Mom and Dad

Self-made doctor and intuitive gentle soul. Both sides of me told me that the world was my oyster, that my dreams would come true. How long did it take that little Star to grow up?

CHAPTER SEVEN 73
Telling My Staff and Colleagues

Stand up, one and all. My staff: Quiet heroines show up despite private heartaches. Now they would have another—

fear for my life and for their jobs. Same goes for my colleagues: Character shines again.

CHAPTER EIGHT 81
Gathering Male Support

Self-made men and rugged individualists. Smart, savvy, and psychologically minded. Solid characters. They know the value of love and humor.

CHAPTER NINE...101
Susan

All the good stuff, plus beauty and humor. No task too big. Loves me and loves her family and friends. A signature laugh filled with mirth. What a woman!

PART THREE: TAKING IT ON

CHAPTER TEN...115
The Options

Cut it, bomb it, freeze it, burn it, starve it. No easy choices, but the atomic bomb looks like a go.

CHAPTER ELEVEN 131
Physical Requirements

Life boiled down to fifteen-minute intervals, diapers, urinals, public restrooms, pocketed pride. I stayed fit with diet, exercise, and meditation. Side effects were draining enough, and I didn't need aggravation from bad habits.

CHAPTER TWELVE..137
   Emotional Tasks

The Serenity Prayer, the Rule of Holes, love and humor. My choice: Survive or live.

CHAPTER THIRTEEN..167
   The Spiritual Challenge

The Great Mystery offers no assurances, justice, reward, or punishment. Prayer is for courage and help, not for outcomes. Santa Claus works for kids, not for grown-ups.

CHAPTER FOURTEEN 191
   Game On

The blow by blow of turning off the gonads, zapping the cancer, and keeping up with my practice, marriage, and personhood. And all the while staring the Grim Reaper in the face.

CHAPTER FIFTEEN 197
   Six-Month Follow-Up

So far, so good. First obstacle cleared, but a lot of marathon left, with many pit stops. Plenty of laughs, too.

CHAPTER SIXTEEN...211
   New Year's Day 2005

Looking decent. Another couple of laboratory hurdles are cleared. Small lifestyle challenges every day.

CHAPTER SEVENTEEN 217
    Blood on the Sheets

Just when my hopes started to rise...Ba da bing! What the hell is this?

PART FOUR: THE MOMENT OF TRUTH

CHAPTER EIGHTEEN...225
    The Moment of Truth

THE trial. Either the Grim Reaper wins, or I win and he is on his way out. Decision: I win!

CHAPTER NINETEEN...231
    Our Dear Little Stone Cottage

So don't think it's over. It ain't ever over. Just the specifics change. The marathon's finish line is the box.

Preface

Prostate cancer suddenly struck from out of nowhere and threatened my life in late summer of 2003. Despite being a psychiatrist with thirty-five years of firsthand clinical and teaching experience, I was first a man—one whose life appeared to be shattered. Terrified and outraged, I was initially flummoxed by the emotional and spiritual crisis that presented me with the challenge of either collapsing in angry despair and dissolution or searching for the lessons while taking cancer on.

As has always been my nature, I went with the latter. Thanks to love from my wife and family, faith in God's mysterious—and at times maddening—universe, and a lot of twisted humor, I appear to have survived. I guess my number hadn't come up for the final call.

At the outset, before knowing any details of the prognosis or outcome, I promised to write about my journey in order to teach. Even if I were going to die, I wanted to do it well and to serve as an example of what men have gone through for years. This book, Ordinary Valor, is the result.

My writing, like my personal growth, has deepened through the life-shaping three-year odyssey of bouncing back from the cancer. The project of journaling my story has been made possible through the loving gift of my wife, who gave unbroken patience. She suspended her leisurely lifestyle and much of our time together in order to allow me the time and space to heal, let alone to write. Despite her misgivings about my being too single-minded and perhaps overworking myself by snatching available hours from leisure time to sit at the computer, she knew I had to do it. She believed in me—and she kept me laughing. With her help, I've avoided getting too serious. That's love. I have deep and endless gratitude for Susan.

My other loved ones, my staff, and my colleagues supported me with their tireless caring and prayers. They tolerated the necessary adjustments to schedules without a smirk or complaint, and their healing energy was an important part of the love that has helped to heal me.

I owe an enormous debt of gratitude to the scientists and clinicians who developed modern treatments for prostate cancer. Had I been born decades earlier, my story would have been different. I hold deep sadness for all the men who have died from metastatic disease—especially those who historically had no effective therapeutic options—and deep sorrow for their wives and children. Special thanks go to my doctor and his colleagues for applying and furthering the contemporary scholarship and techniques of prostate cancer diagnosis and therapy.

My wondrous patients have taught me through the years a knowing that is not found in textbooks or the clinical research of academia. Only now, upon publication, will they learn of my private experience. But along the way, all have implicitly contributed to my professional and personal maturation. They showed me the courage and selflessness necessary to rise above the many heartaches and tragedies that strike in life. All have my utmost admiration and gratitude, rooted in humility. Needless to say, all clinical vignettes and references have been thoroughly disguised so as to protect confidentiality. Composite clinical descriptions allow illustration without disclosure.

I'm grateful to my deceased mother and father, from whom I received undying love and confidence—the basis for my grit and positive attitude. For them, the world was my oyster. Despite growing beyond that fairy tale (immediately accelerated by the cancer crisis), I've kept my unshakable confidence and perseverance.

And in the dark night of my soul, when the Great Mystery seemed especially vexing and when life was appearing both unjust and uncontrollable, God gave me courage and strength. Those, along with making peace with the potholes and rough terrain of my landscape, sustained my morale for staying the course. My intention was to live as fully as I could for whatever time I had.

In short, my faith in divine love and power has had everything to do with my resilience. There are no words to adequately convey my gratitude. I just stay connected.

Laughs, especially those at the most outrageous moments that could have gone the other way, can't be given too much credit. Humor kept me honest and humble—and invigorated.

To craft my journey in the medium of words, Peter Heyrman got me started with his helpful critique. The next stage was to work with the Iowa Writers' Workshop's editorial resource, Iowa Wordwrights. Specifically, I'm grateful to Rebecca Trissler, herself a published author, who explained the fundamentals of how to write a memoir rather than a lecture; in addition, Kathleen Dowling Singh, Ph.D., a clinical colleague and published writer, helped me take it further. The friendly and knowledgeable women at Maine Proofreading contributed the final touches for a clean manuscript. All of their sensitive guidance made possible my giving voice to my experience.

Robert J Mignone, M.D., F.A.P.A.

Introduction

Slowly, gingerly, I lowered myself into the passenger seat. Susan, my wife, had pulled curbside at the hospital discharge exit. She waited patiently for the strap-in ritual which was unusually slow and deliberate on that cool December morning of 2003. I was still nursing my wounded genitals—they had been invaded the day before with the implantation of some hundred-plus radioactive seeds into my prostate. The cancer already should've been on its way to smithereens.

I'd been discharged just an hour previously, immediately upon producing the anxiously awaited golden drops through my catheter. So now it was on to the outpatient X-rays and, finally, home.

I didn't know whether I was more relieved at having cleared the big hurdle or more apprehensive about the follow-through ahead. I tried to relax with deep breaths, but my pulse wouldn't settle down.

With that big intervention behind me, I reflected a moment on the events that had led to the surprising diagnosis, chemical castration, external radiation, and—just 24 hours previously—the implanted radioactive seeds. I'd come through a crisis of far more than a death threat. My view of life and of my priorities had been turned upside down. But discharge day was no time for such introspection. I'd already spent a lot of time meditating in the past four months, and more would follow. Right now, I would do well to concentrate on the moment.

After the prior day's final intervention, the rest of the game was on and I felt like I was at the starting line for the long marathon ahead. My head swirled a bit, and my breathing quickened at such an image, especially since the course was only vaguely mapped out and the finish line unclear.

"Take off, Captain," I barked, trying to appear lighthearted.

"Roger that," Susan retorted, ever ready for a spoof.

As she pulled out into traffic, I made a promise to myself. I knew that the years of recovery that lay before me surely would pose mighty challenges and lessons—maybe no more than those faced by any other man with cancer, but they were big time for me. My life had been on the line for four months and would continue to be for the foreseeable future; that was drama enough. Anyhow, I was determined to make the most of the opportunity and come out of it better off than when I went in. That was my nature. So at that moment, I vowed to use the experience to learn and teach.

"Sweetheart, I'm going to write a book about all this. It probably won't be a thriller. After all, who am I? And who knows what's ahead? But I think telling my story might help other men, let alone their wives...and maybe our sons."

"OK, sweetie, but first let's get you home and settled. Are you OK there?"

"Yes, I'm fine, thanks. It's just that I might as well put this ordeal to some greater good. I'll be damned if I won't come out of this wiser than when I started."

"Of course, Big Doc. But before you save the world, let's get your X-rays or scan or whatever and then take you home to rest while I make you a nice cup of tea and some breakfast."

******

Three years later, I'm still jumping hurdles, still in the race. The familiar cloud of fear hangs far overhead and I try to keep it up there, as does the rest of humanity jogging along with me. Many are limping, but they're still hanging in. I now realize that life will always be like that.

As it has turned out, by some standards my story has been neither glamorous nor amazing, nor has it been raw or juicy. After all, I didn't crash and burn and then rise from the ashes to heroic heights. What I did accomplish was what people do all the time: I faced being turned upside down, gathered myself, and did the best I could to carry on with my life. The lab tests say I'm ahead of the Grim Reaper. That's pretty good. And I grew up a bit. My understanding deepened, and I lost the illusory innocence of a good boy who is rewarded with his prayers coming true, with even getting a pass.

Because my story has been ordinary, I've come to regard my experience as remarkable (even spectacular) because I've seen first hand how it has reflected the marvelous journeys of gazillions of traumatized men and women reeling from crisis while they still worked and loved and managed their lives as best they could – and with only their intimates knowing anything of their heartaches. What courage. They've attended PTA meetings, grooved at concerts, visited families, and showed up at work every day with their game faces on—and never received a medal or a news story. That's amazing. All over the world, people are quietly winning gold medals of the heart. That's the human grit which more than ever brings tears of admiration to my eyes. Celebrities or even unsung heroes may be entertaining and sometimes inspirational, but even more awesome is Everyman's bouncing back. To me, they're all heroes and heroines. I've come to be proud to be one of them.

In short, I lost my innocence and grew up fast. I reinforced my understanding that all we know is worthwhile only if we apply it—and the application requires clearing all the smoke. Only truth works for change. Even world-class scholars of self-care and spirituality can get bogged down looking for pie in the sky, unaware of what they need to actually do in order to grow. I saw my own version of that folly and committed myself to pass it on.

This is not a textbook about prostate cancer or the psychology of coping, although there are thoughts and information about both. And it's not a philosophical discourse about faith or the existence of God, although I talk a lot about my experience of the power of faith. Instead, this is an invitation to walk through one man's journey of coping with the dark night. There have been neither guts nor glory—just everyday triumphs over life's mysterious fragility.

A synopsis might read this way:

Another cancer survival story, this one surprisingly by a man. Good guy who thinks he has it made takes a potentially fatal hit, goes down on one knee, wakes up, and bounces back to do his best because he has balls, faith, a good sense of humor, and a wonderful wife. That's as good as it gets.

Part 1
BOOM

Chapter 1
The Biopsy Result

I barely heard the sound as the concussive wave knocked me back on my heels and stunned all my faculties. The Grim Reaper loomed amongst the swirling shards and debris. My God, is this it?

Late afternoon summer sun streamed through the windows of my second-floor psychiatric consultation room in Sarasota, Florida, giving life to tiny dust particles drifting through slanted beams. The old oak trees outside the tall windows provided shaded privacy, prompting some patients to remark that it felt like we were up in a secret tree house. Upon entering, many commented on what they called casual elegance or a place "just like home." Nearly every newcomer has said something like "Oh, how lovely. This isn't your usual doctor's office." At this point in the day, enough rays pierced through the branches to enter and gently douse everything with a warm glow.

1

Only those patients with a bold sense of humor have teased me about the unruly piles of journals on my desk or the disarray in the bookshelves. I always relished their refreshing candor because it has been a complimentary reflection of their ease. Besides, I've always liked imps.

On that afternoon in August 2003 in Sarasota, Florida, streams of light fell across the rust-colored Oriental rug and mahogany coffee table, enriching the colors and highlighting patterns. Small models of old wooden sailboats and a piece or two of pottery and a crystal on the tabletop provided a pleasant pause for the eye. A box of tissues stood at the ready with the next offering extended through the opening in the top.

My stately grandfather clock ticked its soft, steady rhythm. My very favorite painting in the room, Winslow Homer's *Breezing Up,* depicted three boys sailing away in a catboat, *Glouster,* skippered by the father of the boy sitting in the stern. At the time Homer created it, the Centennial of 1876, the painting was considered one of optimism. One writer stated, "The skipper's son gazing into the illuminate horizon suggests quiet valor, ready cheer and sublime ignorance of bad luck."

There was no trophy wall for diplomas proclaiming my achievements. Those who had not already Googled me or heard about me could read the list of fancy medical degrees and institutions on a one-page listing offered unobtrusively in the waiting room.

My large desk had been my father's consultation desk in his cardiology office. I wondered how many prescriptions and charts written on its leather-bound surface had reflected the bits and pieces of lives, illnesses, and remedies and how many more of life's myriad pains and triumphs had followed that early trail to this desk. In my case alone, the numbers have been in the many tens of

2-11-09

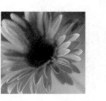

Think of this as a
very large gift well
card. The author is
Dieter He

SIGNED THIS COPY FOR
YOU. TODAY. I AM HOPING
IT WILL BE AN AIDE
IN YOUR FIGHT!

YOUR BROTHER FROM
ANOTHER MOTHER

SR

thousands. Of course, now the leather inlay on top was completely obscured by my journals, prescription pads, pharmaceutical pens, assorted drug samples, and piles of charts. And there was even room for the phone, the dictating machine, a piece of pottery, and pictures of my wife, children, and grandchildren. I knew where everything was in the jumble, but I got relentless teasing from my secretary and occasional patients, for which I was ready with some corny cliché like, "Sign of a great mind." Of course, the dorky comeback just goaded further jibes. Laughter was good here, too.

An antique corner cupboard stood directly behind the desk, which sat on a diagonal facing the doorway in good feng shui fashion. A Chippendale armchair served me behind the desk, and a tailored settee was positioned diagonally in the adjacent corner. Two leather wingback chairs held Mrs. Blanton and me, positioned across from one another, deep in conversation about her life. For me, this time of late afternoon was always a mixture of satisfaction for a day's work well done, a renewed admiration for the human struggle, and a warm sense of imminent closure for the day.

As for Mrs. Blanton, she was her usual gracious self, however pained by talk of her recently deceased husband who had died of lung cancer six weeks ago. His course had been slow and tortuous, but she attended him without fail, right to the end. Hospice provided their saintly succor in the final chapter. From time to time, a tear would trickle down her cheek, to be deftly dabbed with her lace handkerchief.

"Dear Mrs. B., your heart still aches for him, doesn't it?"

"Yes, it does...as you know, Doctor, we were together forty years. He was my everything."

"I do know that. I can only imagine how your heart and soul hurt and how many reminders there are every day."

"Oh yes, even songs on the radio or parts of old movies on the old-movie channel."

"Of course...not to mention that fall is coming up, the time when it all unraveled for you last year, his diagnosis, the start of his treatment. Could you put in words what that brings up so we..."

Suddenly a jolting buzz from the phone intercom cruelly interrupted. I reflexively tightened up, startled. What the hell? It certainly was something big, since Gloria, my secretary, never interrupts. Just a closed door in this place means "Do not disturb for any reason except a real emergency."

This is not good.

Then, hoping my facial expression hadn't conveyed too much alarm or irritation, I offered an apology. "I'm so sorry, Mrs. B., but this doesn't happen except in an emergency. I'm afraid that I must see what it is." She nodded politely and urged me to do so.

As I rose from my chair and walked the few steps to my desk, my head was full of swirling thoughts. My heart rate picked up so that I could feel pulsations in my throat. This must be a patient in acute trouble, an emergency room doctor with a pressing problem, or a loved one in dire straights. Or maybe it was about me.

Oh God, could this be about my recent prostate biopsy?

By that time, I was staring at the blinking red light on my phone, feeling dread in the pit of my stomach and quickening of my breathing. I pushed the button. "I'm sorry to interrupt you, Dr. Mignone, but it's your doctor on the phone. He asked that I buzz you right away."

Something shifted deep inside me. I shivered. My head felt woozy and full of pulsations. I tried to shrug off this

4

feeling with a long, deep breath, but it stuck. This was something I'd tried to push out of my mind for the two weeks since I'd gone in for the prostate stick. As soon as it was over, I'd refused to dwell on the possibilities. In fact, I'd done such a good job of suppression that I'd barely given the pending result any thought at all. Why look for bad news, I'd told Susan. And she was sure the news would be nothing serious. "And if it were, you'll handle it," she said matter-of-factly, expressing confidence without minimizing. So I'd just kept going as usual: up at 5:30 A.M., work out in the gym, in the office by 7:30 or 8:00, and a full practice day; then home with Susan in the evening for dinner on the deck, the evening news, and, finally, journals or my current book, and meditation before bed—same as always. But now, on the other end of this phone line, was the reality of the prostate biopsy result.

Oh, shit. This really can't be good...can't be good. Take a deep breath, Bob.

"Thanks, Gloria. I'll take it from here." I pushed the pause button and steeled myself, feeling furrows dig into my brow. My guts churned. Turning to my patient, I stated, "I'm so sorry, Mrs. B., but I'll have to take this call in the other room. It is indeed urgent. I know this is an imposition, but it just can't be put off." She again nodded and gestured for me to go ahead.

As I slowly walked out of my office and down the hall, my heart kept on pounding as I gasped for breath. My throat and chest tightened.

My urologist is pulling me out of a session with a patient, forcrissake! Damn. This is trouble. This is no courtesy call to give me good news.

Deep inside I wasn't surprised. For months I'd shoved down negative thoughts to beneath the surface of awareness as I tried to ignore some bits of information.

Still, the signs had been there—the extra trips to the toilet in the middle of the night and the mild aches around my groin. All I'd had to do was acknowledge them, but who reads the signs of disaster when the road seems so smooth? Not I. It's as if I had told myself that the crack in the asphalt was just a crack, never a fault line.

Jerk. Boy, oh boy, have you been good at kidding yourself. That's kindly put, I smirked, as I entered the office preoccupied. You know the PSA test read 9.0. You damned well know that the normal range is below 2.0, or maybe 4.0.

In fact, the result had broken through my denial and pushed me into warp speed, at least to the point of arranging a digital rectal exam to search out a prostate mass. The exam results weren't particularly alarming, but that 9.0 still hung there, compelling a biopsy.

The waiting period passed and I felt OK, meaning no new symptoms, so I put the potential bomb in the back of my mind. Besides, I've been an expert at practicing positive thinking (or, more accurately in this case, denial). Indeed, I'd managed to think so positively that I could actually visualize a cancer-free gland.

How's that for a laugh? I smirked again. Big jerk.

And I'd accompanied this optimism with prayer. Each day I prayed for benign prostatic hypertrophy (BPH). That would explain any flow problems.

Sure. What's the expression about a doctor who has himself for a patient having a fool for a doctor, or something like that?

Between the prayers and the visualizations, I'd allowed myself to ignore the seriousness of the problem until this moment when my doctor interrupted a session with my patient.

That's powerful self-deception, Robert, a truly dubious distinction.

Fool.

6

So I arrived at the other office and entered with dread. It was meant to be relaxing and upbeat, with white wicker furniture, brightly colored pillows, dolls, and stuffed animals. Families and kids liked it. That day it felt like a dark cave at the back of which, waiting in ambush, crouched a desk with a blinking red light. And just then, the sun darkened and thunder boomers began to roll. Before nature's special effects amplified my emotions too much, I recalled that Southwest Florida often sees these sudden weather changes this time of year. In fact, the lightning can be fatal.

Easy on the symbolism, my man.

I stood in front of the desk on rubber legs, eyes riveted to the red alert button, and steadied myself by grasping the arm of the desk chair. I slowed my panting to regular breaths and, with my trembling forefinger, tentatively pushed the button that likely would bring life-changing news.

"Hello, Ben. What's up?"

My urologist's voice was somber and caring. "Bob, I'm sorry to intrude like this, but I felt you should know right away." He went on to inform me that my prostate biopsy had come back positive in both lobes, with a Gleason rating of 8 (10 being the worst).

"This is a fairly aggressive cancer, so please get in here ASAP and we can arrange a workup with a total body bone scan, pelvic scan, and more blood tests. Then I can discuss your treatment options with you."

He was being practical, inviting no discussion over the phone.

"Of course," I said automatically.

"I can have our people arrange an appointment with your secretary," he said. His tone was stronger than mere suggestion.

7

"Yes, please do. Thank you, Doctor."

We said our good-byes and I hung up. As I stood there in silence, reality struck.

I wobbled in place, my mind swirling as ideas, intentions, and all other thoughts whipped around like streamers in a high wind. Sweat began to soak through my shirt and broke out on my forehead. Breathing was almost gasping.

I have cancer. Cancer. Cancer. I whispered the words. My God...aggressive and active cancer.... Cancer. My body's eating me alive from the inside. I'm dead. Shit! Shit! Shit!!

Wait a minute—has it spread? Maybe this isn't over yet.

A bit of pressure released as I exhaled through pursed lips.

Just maybe. Gimme any kind of a break here, Lord.

What will I tell Susan? The kids? Should I wait to get the workup? No, she'll want to know now. They'll all want to know. But what do I tell them? I don't even know the facts yet. What a disaster. What a bloody disaster. Oh my God...my God.

My legs gave way, and I slumped back into the wicker desk chair. Once again, I breathed deeply to gather myself. Then all the scary thoughts stopped.

Hold it. Enough is enough for now. I've been a physician for thirty-five years. I know what I have to do. At this moment there's a patient in the other office. She needs my help, and I'm a doctor first. The patient's needs are sacred. Mine can wait. So gather yourself, Robert. First things first. Let's take care of business.

The thunder boomed away, accompanied by a couple of lightning bolts. The heavy drops rattled the windows, and branches tapped them in the blow. How fitting.

I hoisted myself up, set my course back to my office, and left the wicker room to its playthings. With my own cancer deep inside me, I returned to Mrs. Blanton, who had just lost her beloved husband to metastatic lung cancer. And as if that hadn't been enough, it had come on the heels of his two heart attacks, her peptic ulcer, and the near suicide of their grown daughter. I had attended her through much of it. She was a tough and gracious lady. She deserved every bit of my focus, and she was going to get it.

Please, Lord, help me to keep it together. Give me strength to do what I must do.

I needn't have worried about my patient. Upon my reentering the office, she gave me a kind smile. For a moment, it was as if our roles were reversed. I caught my breath, though, and remembered that I was the caregiver. I might not have been able to hold up through an entire hour session, but thankfully we were near the end. I again offered my apologies, said something general about a clinical emergency, and suggested we take up where we left off. My pain was private and not for her to assuage. As we reviewed our work of that day, I was all too aware that the issues we were discussing were the same as those that I was now about to face as a patient. As we finished what remained of her session, it was increasingly obvious to me that I, too, was in for some serious work.

Now there's a brilliant insight, Robert. You probably have no idea of how much, except that it'll be more than you ever had before.

My own ability to cope and heal would be tested to the max. Time to "walk the walk," as they say. In my case, I was fortunate to have clinical experience as a guide. But as I would soon discover, clinical experience goes only so far. I would find inner growth requiring far more knowledge and experience than I had learned from reading and from observing and talking with patients in hospitals and offices.

As she took her leave, I wondered how much Mrs. Blanton had detected. Common sense suggested that she must have noted something, but if she had any inkling of the personal and threatening nature of the call, she didn't let on. The door closed gently behind her and she was gone.

Once again, I was alone with my roaring silence. For a moment, I stared straight ahead, seeing nothing. Then the delayed impact blew the doors off and my floodgates burst. I slumped into my chair, sobbing, as tears poured down my face. Tears flowed for myself and for my wife, children, friends, staff, colleagues, and, yes, my patients.

How broken-hearted will Susan be? Can I still support her? My children and my precious grandchildren will go on without me. I may miss it all. And what about our plans together, Susan and me? And my dreams to teach, my passion for healing others? What of our dear little Rhode Island stone cottage where we've spent vacations? We used to sit on its back porch, have some wine and cheese, and listen to the Tiverton Symphony, our name for the voices of all the birds, tree frogs, and crickets. Are those times over with? Is my practice cooked? What about all my patients? Is all of it finished?

All the images of different parts of my life shattered and slipped away into a numbing dust cloud. I stood up, stepped forward, walked a few steps, and then teetered and fell into the chair that my patient had just occupied. It was as if I'd taken on the patient's role right there in my own office. I wanted to pour out my heart. I wanted to be healed.

Oh Lord, what am I going to do? Help me through this one, please, Lord.

I reached inside to pull it together. Grasping for a handle, I focused on my medical role. I was a doctor. My first instinct was to go on.

But can I? Will I break down in front of the remaining few patients today? Can I stay focused on their troubles and do my patients justice, or would it be more ethical to call off the rest of the afternoon? Either way, should I call Susan right now or wait until I get home?

In that maelstrom came a certain footing, a resolution derived from many years of attending the ill. I would rise above this for now and take care of my patients. Later would be time enough for my own crisis. And, no doubt, it would be a doozy.

Just that rudimentary restructuring gave me enough of a break to collect myself for the moment. As soon as I got the chance at the end of the day, I would come up with my own plan of action. Then I would tell Susan. But for now, I steeled myself. With tears dried, I felt ready.

Focus, Bobby. One step at a time.

Back at my desk, I took a deep breath, exhaled, and reached for my next patient's chart. There I found a small miracle—a yellow Post-it note showing that the patient had called and cancelled. I breathed a prayer of thanks for the brief reprieve.

I knew what I needed in that moment: deep breathing, a clear mind, and some emergency meditation. I talked briefly with God.

Lord, I need your help right now through this storm. Help me keep my focus on their hurt, not mine. I need to stay true to what I do. Stay with me, Lord. I'll get back to you soon, but for now it has to be the next two patients. Help me with the courage to face this. I'm scared as hell, but I have a duty. Help me to carry it out.

I was only forty-five minutes away from—well, from what? I didn't exactly know, but I did realize that I needed to make a short-term plan. I yearned for the day to end

11

within the hour.

Thankfully, I did find the inner resolve to finish with my two remaining patients. They were follow-ups: important, but brief. I bent myself to the task, sweeping aside the wreckage from the bomb that had just gone off.

I had made a judgment call, knowing that the result could work out or go sour. I decided that at least for the next thirty or forty-five minutes, I could focus my mind and empathy on giving care without intrusion from my own crisis. It turned out that I could. Had it been about something even more shattering, like the death or horrible injury to a loved one, I might well not have tried to pull it off. And if the call had come in the morning, requiring that I sit on my disaster all day long, that length of breath holding certainly would have been too much. But as the timing worked out, I was OK with staying the next half hour or so.

The two remaining patients had each suffered a terrible black hole of depression, and one had been suicidal. Mr. Rabinowitz's life had been turned inside out. At one time, he had been at the point of barely making it through the day, but he was courageous and had strong morale. Mrs. Dubinow also had been through her dark night; she too had the grit and resilience to hang in there through the terrible first weeks while the meds began to establish themselves. I prayed with her and for her, debating whether or not to suggest hospitalization. But she emerged from under that cloud to a good place.

Both had worked with me. Our most challenging time was during the first weeks when they had to trust my competence, believe in the treatment, and have the faith and courage to hang in there as the results came slowly.

I also had to believe that I had made the right diagnosis, hadn't missed some important underlying medical condition, and could maintain my own confidence and faith until the clouds parted. Indeed, at first nothing improved as we endured—that has been the course with currently available medications. But over three or four weeks, with psychotherapy, prayer, and medication, each recovered nicely. The lessons we learned together were the commonly known ones of faith, courage, and perseverance. Prayer was for resilience to deal with whatever came along. How prophetic for me. On that particular day, they were in just to touch base, each pleased with their results.

But I knew from clinical experience that their depression could visit again. They were all right now, but how long would that last? Would they keep their balance or fall back into the abyss? We had discussed the possibilities in some detail, so they understood such risks and the signs of trouble. We were at the ready with our response. Needless to say, those questions loomed larger for me than they normally would have. That day, their histories and potentialities, good and bad, struck me with an enormity like none I'd experienced before. Little did they realize how much of their courage I had borrowed.

Over the years, the stories of many patients have both inspired and saddened me. In each were the seeds of learning, not the least of which were from my own moments of doubt about my ability to promote change, the infuriating injustices of life, and the smallness of the contrived focus I had to use in order to address someone's gripping depression or some other psychiatric condition.

In the early moments of reflection after the phone call, I was struck by how much I as a human being had in common with all of those suffering and bewildered souls, and yet how much I differed, for better and worse. Sure, everybody knows about bombs dropping on their lives. I'd witnessed each individual handling them in his or her own way, and I was at times impressed and at times frightened. Now, as my own body was turning against me, I was already trying to find my way through my own dark night. I hoped I could do what my courageous patients had done. At that moment, I was mostly dazed with fear at my life turning upside down.

The thunderstorm had spent itself. The sun was coming back to reclaim the late afternoon, and I could see the parking lot from my window, awash in an inch of water. The drains were teeming, washing away twigs, leaves, and a couple of plastic cup lids.

With privacy for the first time since the bomb struck, I realized with considerable chagrin that, in fact, for years I had not been doing all that I had taught. Embarrassment flushed my face and gooseflesh crept prickly up my neck as I admitted that I'd been caught with my pants down, so to speak. I did not have a doctor and had no regular checkups for anything, let alone for prostate cancer. Hell, I'd been managing my own hypertension. Imagine—I was urging patients to take care of themselves and all the while I didn't even know what my cholesterol or prostate-specific antigen (PSA) values were!

Schmuck.

In fact, if it weren't for the overwhelming and undeniable urge out of nowhere to get a PSA drawn that morning in August 2003, on the way to the hospital, I would likely have continued in my blissful denial, headed for metastatic cancer and death. I'd never gotten routine labs for anything, let alone prostate cancer. I'm "Superdoc." I'd advised others to get them, of course, but not me. So God bailed me out that time by steering my car into the lab parking lot. It literally felt like that. The resulting abnormal PSA blood test marked the beginning of my journey to confront the Great Mystery and stare down the Grim Reaper.

Mortifying. "Schmuck" doesn't begin to say it.

How lucky had I been to have been graced by divine inspiration or His undeniable nudge? It took that much to shake me out of my own subterfuge.

Thank you, God.

Of course I knew that my doubts and fears weren't unique. Neither was my foolish self -neglect. Everyone has known dark nights, and we all know our follies.

This is not the time for bashing yourself, Bob. You can think and learn later. No distractions of "I should've this or could've that." No insults.

So I resisted the temptation to go off on myself, but I did swallow hard as I reminded myself that the details of managing this life have been my own, as has the responsibility. Humility tempered chagrin as I was acutely aware that while all my patients and I have had to face the challenges of bouncing back from traumas, we've done so with both gifts and limitations. At that moment, my shortcomings were needling me, but the imperative for immediate constructive action was trumping them.

I fully realized, as I sat in my favorite office chair reeling from the aftershocks, that I was about to be tested to see what I was made of. So it was high time to apply what I knew and follow it through, no matter the outcome. And if the cancer was localized, maybe I had a chance to live. And if it already had spread? Well, at least I would die trying.

I sank back into my wingback chair as it wrapped around me. I loosened my tie and breathed deep and slow. First, I concentrated on strategy. I would take a walk on the beach where I would figure out how to tell Susan and the children. I could also see an immediate mind-boggling challenge to make sense of this chaos in order to gather myself enough to investigate the workup and treatments…always in the face of the terror of uncertain success.

Talk about crisis management. The action had to start with the here and now because I couldn't afford to distract myself by thinking about a future that might or might not ever arrive.

And, for sure, would come a conversation with The Boss.

Why is this happening to me? Phooey on getting to a mature position of gratitude for the wake-up call. This sucks.

Such a noble concept as personal growth never entered my mind at that early moment. I was just plain pissed, worried, and terrified.

So it's fire department time.

From my safe haven high among the old oaks, all I could see ahead was a jumbled world of crying, worrying, and being turned inside out. I needed to walk and think; I had to get a handle on this. Susan was waiting at home, but before I went to her, I had to gather my thoughts and feelings. I just couldn't come through the doorway a babbling blob.

My next move was clear: go to the beach where I could find solitude for walking meditation. More than ever in my life, I just had to collect myself. I needed to find my center. For that I would need to clear away all bullshit, all platitudes, and any childish magic. Reality was on. I needed real truth and real planning. I headed across the parking lot toward my car.

Part 2

CollectingMyself

Chapter 2
Walking the Beach

I must regroup fast: gather my wits, clear the smoke, and see myself clearly. I can't afford more Superdoc nonsense. Dare to reach out for Susan. And deal with The Boss.

I 've heard that walking is an age-old therapy. Philosophers and religious practitioners have often walked to get the wheels of thought turning and/or to quiet the mind—just what I longed for in that moment. It has been said that walking meditation or reflection takes its centering from both the movement and the solidity of the earth underfoot. Some walk in the woods; others welcome the din of city streets. I knew from experience what I needed and what was readily available where I lived in Sarasota. A few miles away waited the beach, hopefully with the long, flat walking surface of a low tide. I was banking on a quick storm and then clearing weather even though the sky to the west over the Gulf was shades of dark gray.

I strapped myself into the driver's seat, light-headed and in a bit of a fog. Like a robot, I stopped at the lights on South Tamiami Trail, made a right onto Siesta Drive, and followed the road over the Intercoastal Waterway through the village and out to Beach Road, all without any sense of time passing. Thoughts and feelings swirled in the fog and careened off the insides of my skull—worry, fright, resentment, you name it. Ordinarily, I loved looking from the bridge to the north over the waterway to see the boats cruising and the distant two-mile Sarasota condo skyline, but that evening I never even looked. I hardly noticed the lush green tropical foliage lining the North Key Road that hid many of the big homes on the shores of the bay or on the Gulf. Most times I never tired of the view. Moving dreamlike through the village, I took in nothing of the lively restaurants, bars, and shops lining both sides of the bustling street. I managed to avoid hitting jaywalking pedestrians, but I heard none of the jazz, rock, and other sounds of the live bands; no doubt the bars were teeming with laughs, flirtations, and chatter. It was a wonder that I made it through the familiar and scenic route. It may have taken a minute or an hour. The news on the radio was going unheard into the air—I hadn't bothered to turn the car radio off back at the office parking lot—my own news trumped it.

Despite being on automatic pilot, I somehow arrived at the beach and pulled into the parking area strewn (as always) with small drifts of fine white sand. A few scattered puddles from the recent deluge had yet to evaporate. The usual evening walkers were milling about or going to or from the beach. Their numbers were pretty sparse, so I figured most had fled in the face of the precipitous weather change. But some hardy faceless walkers emerged from the pavilion's shelter to return to their treks. I just picked a beach entrance and started walking over the dunes on a wooden slat footpath, going down onto the snowy powder sand and toward the water lying some two hundred yards away.

The beach at Siesta Key was huge. On that evening, moving billows of dark gray washed the sky. A black patch to the southeast was moving inland, carried by the usual August afternoon inshore Gulf breezes. I was probably safe from the lightning bolts known to target bystanders even when the sky overhead looked fairly clear. Our local weathermen were continually warning us in the summer about late afternoon ambushes, especially on beaches and golf courses. Anyway, I might already be dying, so I decided to take my walk then and there.

The gray weather stretched over miles of sand and sea, but due west, over the Gulf, it was clearing. The hugeness of the pastel evening sky made me feel reassuringly small. I could regain some perspective there, with no interruptions or distractions. Even if some friend had hailed me, I wouldn't have heard or noticed. I lucked out on the tide being low because near the water's edge, the footing was sure. I relished the privacy, the calm waters, and the beautiful white beach—and I had the feeling that the perfect setting wasn't random. Small miracles were there to be recognized, even on the brink of a crisis. Gratitude touched my otherwise frantically beating heart as I took off my shoes and felt the warm, wet sand underfoot, noticing my prints being left behind at the water's edge as I strolled. In fact, my surroundings slowly began to come alive.

Admittedly, this wasn't something I did often. Quite the contrary, it was my wife, Susan, who was the beach lover. She usually walked by herself and always found this particular beach to be centering and peaceful; it has been her open-air chapel. Right then arose an irresistible need to follow her example, to share her sacred place. I hoped that even in my state of terror, Siesta Beach would be a source of some measure of solace and energy. Numbness was giving way to fear and worry, so I dearly wanted to be soothed. I dearly wanted to get a grip.

The sand was white and powder-fine, reputedly made from tiny healing crystals. A bronze plaque at the pavilion proclaimed so. People from all over the world have come to Siesta Key looking for a cure by these sands. Susan knew that and came often to walk and absorb the good energy. That evening, I was a believer. My walk there would lead me to the beginning of what I would say to her, of how I would break the news. I hoped that it would be the start of collecting my thoughts for the entire plan of putting back together the pieces.

Even in my turmoil, I smiled to imagine Susan walking gracefully along the water's edge. Salve for a raw wound. She delighted in getting her feet wet, like a wide-eyed giggling child filled with wonderment. In fact, she was an imp about insisting to do so, no matter the temperature of the water, while yours truly got to indulgently carry her shoes. She would place her steps like a dancer and gesture with her arms and hands like a girl obliviously at play. This was all natural, since she always has been without guile. She would direct her beautiful face fully to the setting sun, taking in its energy through every pore. Her fine blonde hair, put up in a top knot, bobbed as she glided along. Her smile and laugh were so distinctive that anyone who knew her would recognize her coming before they could see her. Hers was a mirthful, full-bodied laugh that's at once musical and hearty, infused with unadorned gusto—the kind one feels intimately flattered to be offered. At times it

22

was the squeal of a gleeful woman-child. I could hear it as I walked her path, and it made my heart sing.

Then the poignancy of the moment was pierced with a sudden anguish: I had business to take care of. First, all my cards had to go on the table—a total honesty that I could see for myself. No smoke. That was the only chance I had to find a handle. Because I'm a psychiatrist, one might assume that the process of parsing out a difficult emotional and physical situation would be a natural task. Yes, analysis indeed has been a large part of my professional life for years; I'd done it with many patients and had been involved with analysis and formulation just hours before. But therein lay the catch: The effort had been always for someone else, but now it was my turn. I was the one who had to get past the posturing, the intellectualizing, and all those other slippery defenses of self-deception.

As hard as it was to admit, I had started to acknowledge back at the office that in a few (but important) ways, I'd been conning myself for years. There I was, with my holistic health approach: exercising daily, but carrying thirty pounds of fat; not using nicotine, but unwinding at day's end with a cocktail; using herbs, acupuncture, and healing work, but not even having a doctor.

Sixty-three years old and never had a PSA? Gimmeabreak!

I just had to do better than such self-deception and neglect. I desperately needed to get at the truth, the one inside myself, the hardest one to come by because it would be up to me. Only Susan had the license to confront me from time to time, but I couldn't wait around for her now; I had to peer into my own dark corners. After all, bullshitting myself may have already killed me. Time would soon tell.

So that's the truth you need to get, Bobby. No hiding behind "I'm just human." And certainly no self-bashing.

Your life may hang on this.

The sky began to turn into streaks of oranges, purples, blues, and grays. As I walked along the water's edge, the sun glowed, a huge bright orange ball sinking imperceptibly. Seagulls squawked and dived, vultures searching for food tossed by beach lovers leaving after a day of baking in the hot sun. Hundreds of tiny plovers darted about in perfect unison as if in constant alarm response, but they just couldn't find a consistent route away from their invisible tormenter. Waves had left bits and pieces of dead seaweed to dry and emit their seaside odor. Everything in this vast complexity had its place, its order.

My immersion was at once in the beach world around me, my private thoughts and feelings, and the oneness of it all. A weight sat on my neck and shoulders but did not bow my back as I strolled along the water's edge, zeroing in on my center.

Okay, I've got cancer.

I made myself say it a hundred times.

I've got cancer. I've got cancer. I've got cancer. I've got freaking cancer. Prostate cells running amok, taking over with intent to kill.

Slowly, the dreaded "C" word became life-sized and no longer filled the sky. I was still scared shitless, but at least the cancer became something in my body that I could begin to get my mind around. It sure wasn't going away. Miracles were wonderful, but they were for fairy tales—not for me, not now. I wasn't putting any money on one. All I knew was that I had a killer inside me and that I wasn't going to just lie down and die on the spot. I started to feel a glimmer of pissed-off determination, like I used to feel in the final two minutes of a game's fourth quarter.

With that shift, I could put together a plan. For starters, I needed to learn about this thing. I could see myself pulling books off shelves, reading the basics, talking to colleagues, and hitting the Internet. A picture of the disease, including the most up-to-date information about how to deal with it, would emerge. Any decision would stem from the prognostic implications of the rating scales, the staging, and the therapeutic options with their pros and cons, side effects, and lifestyle implications. That homework would get me to as complete an understanding as was possible. After all, in a crisis like this, with my very life at stake, I wanted every decision to be well informed. I may be a doctor, but I wasn't an expert on prostate cancer. My general knowledge threatened to be a dangerous thing, so the only way to change that was to educate myself.

But wait a minute. Hold it. Stop. What about the emotional side? What about Susan? What about the children?

Oh…Right.

Those were the tough questions.

In just an hour or less, Susan would be with me at home. I would be telling her… what? What should I say? The cold truth? How would the words sound? Would I tremble or mumble or stammer? Would tears flood my words out? Could I actually say that my life was on the line? It had always been "He has cancer" or "She has cancer," but this time the news was all mine, from my own body. It was my ass on the line.

I reminded myself that I wasn't just my own person; I also was someone else's. And that didn't apply just to Susan. There were my sons and stepchildren. How direct and honest must I be with them? And what about close friends, staff, and colleagues? At that moment, I wasn't entirely clear on what I needed to be honest about, let alone with whom and when. After all, I didn't have all the information.

Is the cancer localized or metastasized? Will I survive

25

with treatment? And if so, with what quality of life? Or am I already walking dead? I won't know that for a while.

Cancer confined to the prostate gland itself is potentially curable, but if it spreads to other parts of the body, it's not. Lights out. And in the meantime, Susan and I will have to live with a sword dangling over our heads. *So there's no truth to tell*, I proffered half-heartedly, trying to wiggle off the hook.

How can they be burdened before the truth is clear? I don't want to needlessly worry them.

But then came to mind my wife—the real Susan, not the one I'd contrived in my foggy defenses. She certainly knew enough about how cancer worked. She already knew about the PSA result and that I'd had the biopsy. If I held back from her, she wouldn't be fooled. I would just be trying to fool myself.

I watched the very mechanism of my avoidance: keep analyzing and never have to act emotionally. What she knew or couldn't yet know wasn't the point; she deserved to know now. Because she was my wife and because we were who we were to each other, she should know all of this from the start—the frightening unknown and the unfolding of the answers. I had to take the dare to put truth and her love above my own Superdoc nonsense. That was the only way it could be between two people who loved each other, so I vowed that she would know what I knew as soon as I learned it.

I'll give her every bit of reassurance that I can, I said to myself with forced bravado. I'll do the right thing. And I'll let myself be vulnerable. I will not drop the ball. That's a promise.

Hold up, my friend. What are you smoking? Do you really think she'll assume anything else? There you go again. You're whistling in the dark again with your damned doctor intellectualizing. This is not just about doing the right thing. Reassurance also is not the main issue. This is not a brain thing—it's a heart thing. The point of telling her now is to allow her to love you in the way she would want to. Her sharing all of this with you is a way for her to give you her gift of compassion and loving support. Remember the two-way street?

In a way, this was a simple reapplication of Sutton's Law. Willie Sutton was a bank robber who, when asked why he robbed banks, allegedly replied: "Because that's where the money is." In other words, don't screw around; get your target and go straight for it. So to get grounded and set for crisis response, I went for the truth. But also I needed support, tenderness, and care, as well as someone who could tell me the truth. In a word: love.

When I need love, I go where the love is. That's Sutton's Law.

I didn't need to be told where that was. Fourteen years before, I had found the wellspring for love in my wife, Susan. Also there were the kids—my two boys and my two stepchildren—as well as friends, colleagues, and coworkers. It wasn't that I didn't know where to go. The question was: Did I dare go there? Could Superdoc, the almighty who needs nothing and cares for all, bring himself to go there?

By the time I arrived that far in my thinking; I had turned around to begin the long amble back down the beach. The sky behind me to the northwest had cleared to a rosy color with peach streaks. The dark patch ahead of me by now had moved east, nearly out of my line of sight and hidden by the spiky rows of tall condos strung out along the beach to the south. I looked for my footprints to retrace, but they'd been washed away. The gulls of different colors and sizes were still in the hunt for the last scraps. Their sculpted forms swooped gracefully, determined and relentless; they squawked, postured, bowed, scurried, and maneuvered to maintain communication.

Sooner or later, each found what it needed to survive: a bit of sandwich, a corn chip, a piece of cookie. Then they strutted, showing off the prize dangling from their beaks. The sky was becoming a glowing red-orange. I turned around to behold the bright orange ball settling down for the day, bisected against the horizon. The sand underfoot was cooling as I cut new prints. My step had more energy, and I picked up the pace without thinking about it. The Gulf waves gently caressed the shore, rolling in new shells for the self-sustaining collection.

And now came the time to deal with the Other One— The Boss. I raised my eyes to the evening sky and took in the sunset.

And now for You, God. What's up with this? Is this some kind of punishment or dirty trick? Are you trying to kill me for not paying attention? Or are You just not paying attention here? This is me, Bobby, and it's not supposed to be happening, not here, not now, not when I'm just getting to the top of my game. Why screw it all up now?

I kept looking at the sky. I went on.

I don't deserve this. I'm a good guy, damn it. I do good things for people. I don't fool around or hurt people, and I love my wife and family. What the hell has justified this? I pray for reasonable things. I'm not just looking for magic. So where are You? Is this supposed to be one of those life lessons? As the kids say, "Shit happens to the good guys, too." Right? Is it the one about learning in the school of hard knocks? Do I really need this now?

Why the Job deal? I have faith. I pray every day. What about co-creation? Positive intention? Doesn't being loving and kind count for anything? My intentions are clear and good. Isn't that what the New Agers talk about? Creating good energy that comes back in kind? Co-creating? Or is that more bullshit? Praying for outcomes obviously doesn't work. If somehow I didn't learn to believe that from thousands of suffering and dying patients, I sure know it now. So is faith, like Freud said, just pablum for the masses? Or was I praying for the wrong things? I help my suffering patients every day. And now I get repaid with suffering. Is there no justice? Talk to me.

I kept my pace and focus.

OK, maybe it's my turn. Maybe I have to learn what everyone knows about life, this time through my own experience. Like it or lump it, life's a big fat mystery. As for fairness, accountability, reward, or predictability, forget about it. Maybe I have been expecting magic.

It's only what I make of it, how I take the hits. There's that big unknown plan, which has more undeserved tragedy and evil behavior than I've cared to admit, but somehow that fits. Right? No sense and no control—part of the Great Mystery.

At this point, my heart rate was slowing down and the heat in my head was cooling off. The orange ball had nearly disappeared.

Well, Boss, You sure have upped the ante. Lesson or no lesson, growth or whatever, this sucks. Stick with me, please, Dear Friend. We'll weather all this together and find out what the story is. I'm plenty mad and scared right now, but I need You more than ever. I'm not going anywhere. We'll be back in touch as soon as possible. I have a lot of stuff to sort out—as if You don't already know that. But now...

******

It was time to start dealing with my family. It was time to tell Susan, who was waiting at home, fifteen minutes away. I took one last look at the beach panorama, shuddered at such beauty never before appreciated to this degree, and headed for the wooden walkway that lifted me over the dunes and down to the parking lot.

Chapter 3

The Ride Home

On my way to tell Susan, I lost myself in reverie about what may be the last delicious memories of our happy homes. Next might come nursing homes.

As I settled into my car and started out of the parking lot, I drove through a couple of remaining puddles in low-lying spots, hearing the quiet slosh and feeling the cleared ocean air through open windows. I wanted to hear and smell everything. Who knew how much time I had left to do so? I inhaled chi—or life force—down into the depths of my lungs through my nose and exhaled through pursed lips to make a wind sound. I'd always centered with that maneuver.

I planned to reflect on my beach walk while I headed south on Midnight Pass Road toward home. I decided then and there that it should forever be called "The Walk" because it had been like an accelerated mini-passage. I smiled at the thought of having shifted a bit from an immature tantrum to a more grown-up response. It actually felt good to begin to get to the truth and face it straight on. In fact, I didn't feel quite so shattered anymore. Yes, I'd taken a body blow, and it seemed like the last thing on earth I'd needed. I was trembling with fear inside, but I was on my feet, already determined to conjure up the resolve to take it on with faith and love—from Susan, my children, and God. At least I was starting to feel a little more in the driver's seat, though still plenty scared and pissed. But at least I'd established a beginning. Of course the awareness was well and good, but the real question—the one that would determine a lot about whether I would live or die— was could I follow through? Did I have what it takes to make good on insights? If so, I had a chance; if not, all the thinking that late afternoon after the call would have been mere psychobabble.

So I came up with take-home lessons that I recorded for future reference when inevitably I would be shaky. I pulled over into the parking area of one of the many condos lining the beach road, found a piece of paper lying on the front seat, and scribbled down the ideas using one of the ubiquitous drug company pens found everywhere (in my shirt pockets, on the car dashboard, and so on).

Yes, I needed my tantrum, and I needed to go through the gymnastics of denial and rationalization. Fine. I got it out of my system. Fast. Then I at least started to grow up. Real fast. I stopped bullshitting myself and cleared the smoke. I got to as much of the truth as I possibly could. Then and only then was I free to reach out to love. And only then could I get my brain in gear to use what I knew, and to start learning and applying what I needed.

Lock that in your archives, Robert.

In that honest and centered place, I'd lost my

innocence. I'd had a crash course about what I'd taught others—a mature sense of the Serenity Prayer and a deepening faith. Santa is good only for kids at Christmas. After my wake-up call, I'd begun (like a grown-up) to face the mystery of why bad things suddenly happen without warning or apparent justice. I didn't like it one bit, but reality was the priority. It was a tough way to be reminded that life surely can come apart at the seams in an instant, with no sane reason. But what awareness comes easy? And who doesn't know that?

It was clear on the drive home that I either cave in or deal and I damned well wasn't going to cave in, so I wrote the note for reference in the days and weeks ahead. There surely would be lots of researching, thinking, and meditating, all of which required my getting on course and staying there. This cancer was going to be what I made of it—ordeal or wake-up call, or both.

Huge challenge, Bobby.

Right there behind the wheel, I started to pray for courage and strength to do my best.

I pulled back out into the flow of traffic toward home and noticed a car ahead of me with a bumper sticker: **Jesus Saves.** I snorted and offered a different one: **Help Jesus Save You: Sit Down and Shut Up, Dial Up, and Grow Up.**

******

The surreal drive from the beach to our house followed the two-lane road that ran southward down the middle of southern Siesta Key. On either side, substantial homes sat behind walls, and lush tropical landscaping burst out of gardens. All sorts of palms, tall and bushy, overflowed; live oaks and cypress trees lined the street, often arching from each side to embrace in a canopy.

That evening every tree, bush, driveway entrance, and patch of gray sky above the canopy was filled with life. I was heading south, following the tail of the vanishing storm. I was on my way to Susan, but I was so lost in reverie that it was like I was somewhere else. Arrival was five minutes away but was light years away. Exquisitely vivid daydreams distracted me from my destination's terrifying business.

Susan was waiting my arrival in our sanctuary.

What does a dying man think about on his way to his own funeral? For me, it's my wife, my home, and my kids. I want to savor every memory I can. Who knows how much longer I'll have them in this life?

So I wasn't merely trying to distract myself by immersion in delicious scenes and vignettes. I was grasping to hold onto them, to embrace and incorporate as much as I could—in fact, I damned well was going to savor every morsel. So with angry defiance and near-frantic desperation, I gorged on memories. I nearly burst with wanting to eat, drink, hug, kiss, tease, laugh, cry, make love, rage, howl, run, and do whatever else I could to cram a lifetime into the last few minutes before I laid the bomb on Susan.

In fact, I was so absorbed that I barely maintained enough presence of mind to avoid sideswiping a bicyclist on the roadside. My alarm response flooded for a few minutes, sending my cardiovascular system into flushed palpitations before I could calm down. By that time I was in the south village, with shops on my left and waterfront short-term rentals on my right. I was probably going slower than the 25 mph limit, but the few fellow drivers didn't seem to mind what must have been a creeping pace. Anyway, if they had, I wouldn't have noticed.

One after another our magical homes crossed my mind: candlelit holidays, festive birthdays, and exuberant grandchildren romping in the pool or scratching the surface of some antique with a small model car. Our sanctuaries changed from an eighteenth-century Federal (before moving to Florida) to an old Florida tin-roofed house on a river replete with old oak hammocks and real live gators. The incredulous kids teased us about moving from Masterpiece Theater to the Wild Kingdom. What wondrous soil for the roots of our marriage—rich, juicy, and nutritious. Then on to an old Ringling-style Italianate mansion in Sarasota that had its own magic, like a movie set out of the 1930s. And finally the big West Indies home on Siesta Key to which I was headed.

The scenes that flashed weren't about Susan's brilliant taste and decoration. They were about the humanness that filled each of the places—the warmth, the hundreds of lit candles, the laughing, crying, making love, thinking, working.

Were all those magic moments gone from my life? For that matter, how much of my life is left?

Tears welled up and made it difficult to see to drive. I didn't know whether to pound on my steering wheel or bawl. I almost had to pull over, but I managed to extract a handkerchief from my back pocket and mopped up enough to keep driving. And I quickly thought better of busting up my steering wheel. Home wasn't much farther down the road.

Did I take all those times for granted? Did I thank God enough for the bounty? No. Was I appreciative enough of Susan bringing into my life her unique mixture of classy taste and earthy humor? Probably not. Not enough, anyway. There couldn't be enough of that.

Was I finished with homes as we've known them?

Would it be nursing homes from now on? Or would it be a hospital bed with hanging intravenous poles? Or—and here's a lovely thought—maybe even hospice?

I was nearly at the entrance. No more fantasizing about what might have been my prematurely final chapters of healthy happiness. Here was present reality, a few hundred yards away on the right.

How will Susan take this? Will she burst into tears? If she does, it'll go right through my heart and I'll lose it big time. For that matter, can I tell her straight out?

Palpitations rose in my throat and I started to choke up.

Oh, shit. This won't do. You can't lose it, baby. Chill. Stay focused on business.

Just then, out of the corner of my right eye, I spotted the trunk of a car backing out of a neighbor's driveway into the street just ahead of me. I slammed on the brakes in time, but I still got the finger and a string of curses that I couldn't hear because of the closed car windows. I shrugged sheepishly in feigned apology. What a waste of passion.

The scene struck me as so ludicrous that I didn't have to calm myself. It was but a silly sneeze in the course of a profoundly meaningful mission—asking Susan to share my possible death sentence and her earthquake. Then the white brick pillars marking the entrance to our driveway came into view.

Okay, Bob. Time's up. You're on. Get ready, sweetheart.

As I turned left into the drive, I anticipated the lush foliage and our majestic West Indies house built up over flood level, with balcony decks front and rear. I reached inside for the familiar flutter of delight upon coming home. However, a coldness in my chest snuffed the fondness as I wondered whether all the wondrous memories were about to be shattered. Or if I were lucky, maybe it would be more like shaken.

Am I going to be able to continue carrying this place, or will we be forced to sell? Stop. Let's not go there. This is home. Take it step by step, one minute at a time.

I pulled in through the entrance columns and drove slowly around the circular shell driveway up to the front entrance, acutely aware of all my senses. The tires crunched the shells, and a subtle aroma wafted from the bountiful orange and grapefruit trees in the center lawn circumscribed by the drive. The sprinkler system spouts sputtered and spit their desperately vital sustenance to the lush plantings. The greens of the palms and foliage were especially verdant, and the reds, oranges, and yellows of the bromeliads were proudly brilliant; even the delicate moss hung gracefully like lace from the oak branches, as if carefully draped there by angels. In the distance the drone of a lawn mower indicated attention to someone's lawn. Or maybe it was somebody blowing leaves and debris from one spot to another, and I smirked at one of my pet peeves.

A large white heron gracefully high-stepped in slow motion through a side garden and went off toward the lagoon side of the house. If it couldn't find little lizards, then small fish would do. This evening its carriage was especially majestic.

Tears were running down my cheeks. The beauty of it all piqued my sense of irony. How delicious was every moment, every element of life—every plant, stone, shell, brick, animal, or piece of debris; every sound, every smell, every texture—and how fragile. My sobs were building.

This won't do, Bobby. Not that there's anything wrong with overflowing, but it'll prevent you from telling Susan. You will NOT turn into a puddle of tears. That's just not going to happen here. She would feel compelled to gather herself tightly to compensate for your falling apart. Not

37

good for either of us. And it would abort the mission. No way is that going to happen. So, my man, get a grip, take a deep breath, and step up.

I did so, drying my face, exhaling, and focusing on my promise. I got out of my car and walked in a daze up the brick entrance walk between the ground foliage that Zak and I had broken our backs to install—not once, but three times! I grinned, relieved to get my mind on something else, if even for a second. But soon I was at the large paneled door.

Chapter 4

Breaking the News to Susan

Trembling and sweating, I eked out the "C" word. She pulled me to her breast. Then she cracked me up. Guffaws and tears, doubts and promises. The first big hurdle was cleared.

The large brass handle of glass-paneled double French doors was cool to my tentative grasp. The ordinarily fluid opening swing resisted my pull but finally yielded. I stepped into my foyer like I was trespassing.

Should I sneak upstairs and then find Susan? Or maybe she would be out for a walk.

Coward.

Or should I fake my usual self, hailing her as I entered and then bounding up the steps to greet her? Oh, come on, we just went through this. Just do it.

So I cleared my throat, mustered as much chi in my chest as I could, and called out something short and familiar like "Suzy, I'm home."

Since sound reverberates in the lofty interior, I assumed that she had heard me. I grasped the railing and started up. My wooden legs trudged, one by one. Twenty-five feet overhead in the atrium loomed the big brass chandelier constrained by one thin chain from bashing in my skull. I noticed and grinned.

Come on, Bob, do this thing.

Susan heard the leaden thuds of my footsteps and came to greet me as usual, but this time she detected the different pace and energy. I hadn't given her my usual hearty greeting or banter, and I sure wasn't bounding. So she started down the first few stairs and held out her arms. She was more beautiful than ever in her white linen top and three-quarter-length pants; her blonde hair was in a single braid in back, and she wore a funky handmade silver necklace with an amethyst pendant. Her beautiful face had a puzzled and even apprehensive look. Her throaty voice was uncharacteristically hesitant.

"What's the matter, sweetheart, don't you feel well? Has something happened?"

"No and yes…we need to talk."

"Oh my God, come up here and tell me. You look like something bad has happened." She took my trembling arm and gently but firmly led me for the last few steps.

"It has, but let's sit down…"

Then she took my hand, which by that time was moist. We walked together in silence over to the sofa in the living room, the place where we sat at the end of each day to reconnect and chat about the day's events. This would be the chat to end all chats. I hardly noticed the dark pink-streaked sky through the French doors that opened out onto the deck overlooking the languid water, and I barely glanced at the fresh flowers she had cut from the garden and lovingly placed in a vase on the coffee table in front of the sofa where we always sat at day's end. I didn't even remark on her new manicure or hair coloring.

I certainly had no banter, no jokes, and no inquiries about what she did with her day or what she might have heard that day from any of the kids. Instead, I sat down and then sank slowly into the sofa, exhaling loudly as I unfolded. So did Susan, right beside me. By this time she was waiting eagerly, if not apprehensively, for what I had to tell her that was so out of the ordinary. I had all I could do to stay with my plan that I devised on the beach and reinforced in the car.

Just out with it. She can take anything. Let her love you.

I started to speak but found my mouth was dry as straw. I pressed on. "The biopsy came back," I whispered. "It was positive. It's prostate cancer...aggressive. God only knows if it is local or has spread, so the prognosis is up in the air. It could be lethal or curable. I don't know if I'll live or die. But you can be sure that I'll get the workup and find out. We'll know more in a few weeks."

She reached over and touched my cheek. "Shush," she was cooing through pursed lips.

She didn't need to hear any more reassurance. She folded her arms around me in a long hug. With both surprise and relief, I settled into her bosom gratefully, with ease. For some reason, I'd wondered if I could ever touch anything again. Without my even knowing it, the news had distanced me that much from my normal world. Susan pulled me back just by holding me. I could feel her breathing, her heart pounding. And, as always, I noticed that sweet smell of the skin about her face and neck, soft and velvety like a baby's. Often I called her "Velvet." She stroked my forehead with a soft but definite caress. My racing heart slowed, and my trembling stopped.

41

How defensive I'd been. How taut my muscles had become. Now that was dissipated. We were a team facing a challenge. By this time we were both weeping, me especially—I tend to be the slobbery one.

"We'll do whatever we have to do to handle whatever comes," she said. "I know this will be all right. You're not going to die from this. I just know it. And of course you'll do it right. When have you done anything otherwise?"

She squeezed my hand. It was only after she said this that the apprehension began to cloud her beautiful face. Her million-dollar smile tightened and her eyes again grew moist. Then she shrugged. "Shit happens." I had to laugh through the tears.

She went on. "OK, this time it's prostate cancer. When will my time come? And for what? Breast cancer? A stroke? This is part of life. Like you always say, 'Into every life some turds must fall.' Our job is to deal with it. Love will see us through this."

It struck me that, knowingly or unknowingly, she was playing back to me some of my own thinking. But now the action was live and painfully personal. Anyhow, she herself knew what was called for and was right on the mark. She kept the focus on my pain, not hers, at least for the time being. I hoped she wasn't denying her pain to spare me. I wanted her to be honest for her own sake and said so.

"No, I'm not making too little of my feelings. I know in my heart that you'll be all right. This will not kill you. It will be a pain in the ass. And of course you're scared. Who isn't? After all, it's your life at stake, here, sweetheart. I just know you'll be okay."

She seemed centered and sure, not shaken and hiding, and I well knew her strong intuition and fearless courage. She's always been an old soul. I knew she genuinely believed what she was saying. At that moment I needed

42

some of that.

From there we talked and wept, wept and talked. We reminisced about our life together, cherishing it, nodding and smiling.

"Remember the vacations on Nantucket," I mused, "riding the bike trails and walking the beaches? We rode the entire island many times and never came within fifteen feet of a passing car. And remember we were there on 9/11? I was at the bakery counter buying chocolate chip cookies for us when a lady next to me in line said her daughter in New York had just called on her cell phone to say that a plane had just struck the World Trade Center. She, I, and the few others in line assumed that it had been a small prop plane gone astray. And then I came out to the car to tell you, and it dawned on us that it could be something more. Trying not to catastrophize, we raced back to our rental cottage and watched the horror unfold on TV in front of our eyes. And then remember the terrifying realization that Polly's husband--our son-in-law, Jon-- worked at the top of the building? What a relief to learn two hours later that he was safe, having taken a later train into the city, thanks to Monday night football the evening before." We both shuddered and exhaled.

Talk about fragility.

Even as that horror and terror struck the world, my own mortality never really hit home, even in the face of that out-of-the-blue unfathomable intrusion. We felt terrible for the victims, bewildered at the senselessness of it, and disillusioned that such things could happen. But in my own egocentric world, the Great Mystery didn't deeply touch me until I was on the block with cancer.

Was everyone moved only by imminent personal assault?

Susan then changed the subject. "And the time in

Vancouver where we enjoyed that once-in-a-lifetime chance of five straight days of sunshine?" We went on about that a bit, until I recalled a Chinese pavilion in Vancouver's China Town and its garden where she spontaneously did tai chi under the roof of a small pagoda perched on an arm of land out in the middle of a pond. I wept for the beauty of it

"Oh for God's sake, you cry at anything," she teased with her signature impishness.

There've been many more fond memories, now bittersweet. Would there ever be more? Or was that it for our travels and our shared times? Don't go there, Bob.

"Will our future times be in hospitals and nursing homes? Maybe the most we'll travel is from home to the doctor's office and then to the lab and then back home. Some round trip, eh?"

"Easy, big guy. Don't get too precious here. We'll do what we must, but this is not the end. This will not kill you. A big pain in the ass? Yes, but we'll see our grandchildren grow up."

I knew she was neither quashing sharing nor resorting to pie in the sky. She used humor to help me stay on course to do what I needed to do, including being honest with my feelings. She well knew that lapsing into worst case scenario was its own defense. Also, she was not a denier by nature; it was just not the time she chose to vent her own pain. She put mine first.

That's some empathy and some love. This woman knows me and knows how to help me avoid losing my focus.

I gradually felt myself settling, but I was still shaken. No doubt Susan was, too, but she kept her pain in the background, holding mine front and center. Like I said, I hoped it wasn't a false bravado.

With all this heart-wrenching reminiscing going on, Susan still had it in her to pull "a Susan." She got up from the couch, excused herself, went into the kitchen, opened the refrigerator, and—in plain view from where I sat in the living room—took out a bottle of champagne. With her one-in-a-million impish smile, she waved it playfully and announced, "You know, sometimes you just have to say, "What the f..."

I roared with peals of laughter and relief. What an icebreaker.

Leave it to her. Perfect timing. A natural comedienne who knows just when and how to lighten the mood. And never trivialize.

So we sipped champagne through our tears and chuckles. We bantered about my life insurance making her a richer widow than a live doctor's wife and about needing to make sure my will was up to date. My tears tasted salty in the laughter.

"Oh, dahl...ing," she said, feigning affection, "before you die, would you mind pouring me another glass?"

Thank God for Susan.

Then it was planning and strategy time. We both knew instinctively that we had to be committed to staying informed and positive. Susan knew it was important for me to say all this out loud. I guess doing so endowed all our intentions and hopes with the greater power of personal commitment. She may not have needed it, but apparently I did.

"OK, you go ahead and do your thing with looking up the information. You know how well you can research anything, especially in medicine. Learn all about this prostate thing. Tell me what I need to know, but not all the details. Those are for you and your doctor. For me, I want

45

to know what your treatments are going to be and what we can expect for side effects. We'll do whatever is needed. I know you'll come out of this just fine."

There's her conviction again. Does she have some direct line to the Almighty?

"Oh, so now you admit you're intuitive," I quipped. "No more teasing me about 'Woo Woo.'"

"Oh no, I'll never stop that. But yes, I do know you'll be OK. This is not our last call. This is just a big pain in the...ah...prostate."

******

This certainly was the most difficult life crisis either of us had handled, but we weren't babes in the woods. Both of us had lost parents: I had lost both; she had lost her father, and her mother was ailing with severe emphysema, surviving with the long green tube. In the early 1990s, Susan had also lost a brother to cancer. Before we found each other, both of us had been through divorces, surviving the difficulties of split parenthood. At one point in the late 1990s, I'd been the board chairman of a charter school, and when it collapsed financially, I was left holding the bag—I even had to file Chapter 13 as they went after deep pockets regardless of merit. But we'd gotten through that as well. So we weren't strangers to heartaches. We'd known them alone and together. Together was better.

This time, my own death was staring me in the face. I had to confront the mystery of why bad things happen to the good guys. As for Susan, she was coping with the possibility of her life turning upside down. But it was some time before she brought that out in the open. It was her intuitive belief and her loving empathy, rather than avoidance, that put my immediate needs above hers. But I couldn't help continually worrying about whether she was stuffing her own important pain.

Nonetheless, she gave me license to indulge my emotions and thoughts. I knew that was self-centered, but with her permission and encouragement, I let it rip some more. "I'm bloody outraged and I'm scared as hell. But I will handle this colossal piece of merde. I will do what I have to do, for me, for us. I will not tank on you. I promise. I'm already up to the plate."

"I wouldn't expect anything less."

Once again she'd touched my heart. I wept some more.

"Thank you for loving me."

"Sure, sweetheart, anything for your bucks."

"No, I'm serious."

"Of course, my darling." Then serious and weepy, she said, "You're my life, too." She hugged me big time.

Finally, after having bared my soul to Susan, I was ready to call my sons—Marcus in Connecticut and Paul in Boston—and my stepdaughter, Polly, in New Jersey. The lack of face-to-face conversation would cut both ways. I might be able to maintain more composure, for what that would be worth, but I also couldn't connect emotionally as effectively as I could in person. But since all of them but Zak, my stepson living in Sarasota, were over a thousand miles away, there was no choice. Only Zak would be told face-to-face.

Chapter 5
Telling the Children

Marcus, Paul, Polly, and Zak. Don't just inform; ask to be loved. Easier said than dared.

I couldn't recall whether I called Marcus or Paul first. No matter, because there wouldn't have been a reason either way. Both have become mature husbands, good fathers, and extraordinarily successful entrepreneurs. Each has developed his own personality, sharing only certain elements with one another and with me. Of course that would be no surprise—especially to Susan who often teased, "You're all Mignones...smart, hard working, never quitting, climbing on no one's shoulders. Know-it-alls. Kings of the hill, all three of you. Only Marcus takes care of himself. You and Paul? Well, so far it doesn't look like you, at least, are getting away with it." Anyhow, your family loves you. So do your friends."

Since my folly in stumbling onto the diagnosis of my

cancer seemingly by dumb luck, Susan has had the grace to avoid an "I told you so" regarding my not taking care of myself enough in some areas. She certainly heard me admit as much during our conversation earlier that evening when I told her about my thoughts since the cancer phone call. I'd also mentioned that I feared for Paul's avoidance of doctors and wanted him to learn from my mistake. But there was no call for preaching at that moment; he would come to his own awakening about self-care. I just wanted him to get there sooner than I had.

When I left Massachusetts for Florida with my new bride, the boys were in their early twenties, already men on their way to adult lives. The reasons for my relocation had nothing to do with them; in fact, I decided to go despite wanting to remain near them. Susan loathed cold winters, and I'd "been there, done that" in the regional psychiatric scene, at least insofar as I was willing to deal with the cliques, circles, and networks. Also, managed care was already creeping into liberal Massachusetts and growing fast. I saw it as a cancer to quality private practice, at least the kind I practiced.

So I longed for new professional possibilities. I welcomed a new start to open up new areas of interest in psychiatry and to further develop the concept of a multi-specialty mental health group, perhaps in multiple locations. I also wanted a sunny environment for Susan. We headed for a place that was nothing but possibilities— Southwest Florida. For one thing, there was little psychiatric development, at least compared to what I'd known in greater Boston.

The only heartache in moving to Florida was my removal from my sons' daily lives. I'd been their coach and their devoted male figure despite a killer practice schedule. Since the move to Florida, however, I no longer saw them daily and was no longer intertwined in their lives.

In fact, for the past twelve years the occasional phone call had had to suffice. A visit every summer had barely cut it with my grandchildren, who knew me only as an old guy who (with his wife) visited twice a year, coming from someplace far away called Florida. This limited intimacy has been for me a source of regret and sadness, especially regarding my part. I had left town and tended to stay in touch only sparingly, especially as the years went by and my life became very busy. Past attempts to apologize for my shortcomings as an overly busy father through their teen years had been met with brush-offs like "Hey, that's all behind us. You did the best you could then. We had our problems, too." There was some wisdom in that, but the subtle pattern of distance had grown over time. Maybe telling them about my cancer and possible death would shake up the three of us.

To say the least, then, the calls I was about to make were going to be most unusual. For one thing, it was the first time we would be sharing the possibility of one of our deaths. Secondly, I was calling in the midst of the storm for support, not after the fact to merely inform.

Walking over to the phone in our kitchen to make the call, I gasped at the memory of my own father's death. My chest swelled and a lump rose in my throat. I paused and took myself back in memory to New Haven, 1983, with my two sons at each of my sides, poised to enter for the first time the room in the funeral home where Dad lay in an open casket. I wept at seeing his body, but both Marcus and Paul were fixed on helping to hold me together, each taking one of my arms as if holding me up. At the moment of no return, we looked at one another. I saw right down into their stalwart hearts, and thus strengthened, I stepped forward into pain. Like three soldiers, we marched into the

51

room up to his coffin to say good-bye. Dad's spirit must have been proud. I sure was—and grateful ever since.

A deep breath and I'm back in the kitchen on Siesta Key. I pushed back the few tears remaining from the memory of my sons supporting me back then and dialed first one and then the other. My message was essentially the same to both despite knowing that, as distinct individuals, each would react internally in his own way. Maybe I was still doing my version of perpetuating the subtle reticence. But because I wasn't hoping for any deep discussion at that moment, I just wanted to inform them and then feel a caring connection. I thought anything more would have sounded like psychobabble. So it went something like this: "Son, I have potentially bad news, so sit down and prepare yourself. I have prostate cancer. I don't know if I caught it in time; only the workup will tell. I'm OK for now. I'm going to see what the details are and decide on treatments. Of course I'll keep you included along the way."

I'm sure my attempt to be straightforward, without sounding nonchalant, was transparent, but neither of them called me on it at that moment. I assured them that I was taking the whole thing seriously and that my approach would be constructive. "I'm going to tackle this straight-on. I will not go down and I will not tank," I said to both of them.

When I looked back on that posturing, I could have gagged.

Who the hell did you think you were fooling?

Marcus and Paul must have as well. Initially, I barely gave either one a chance to express much of their concern beyond expressions of surprise, reassurance, and promises of loyalty. It was clear to all of us as we talked later after the fact that it had been just a variation of the "Big Daddy" camouflage they had come to know. Both of my guys immediately read right through that. They told me later that they knew my assurances were more for me than for them; they weren't fooled. Both are strong grown men who have weathered their own storms and have found their own wisdom.

So despite myself, each gave me love and support. And even in the face of my half-assed attempt to reach out, I was aware of loosening up on my bionic nonsense. I consciously avoided trashing myself for the brave front. All I could do was do better next time, though it better not be another death threat.

"You'll beat this, Dad," Marcus said confidently. "After all, you're a Mignone."

Paul also expressed his assurances and, like Marcus, asked, "Do you need anything? What can I do?"

"Just be there, thanks. Love your family and relish every minute. If I need something, I'll definitely ask. Thanks again. I love you, too."

******

Now to tell my stepchildren, Zak and Polly. I could talk to Zak face-to-face because at the time he lived in our house in an apartment on the ground floor. I walked down the stairs to his apartment and asked him to sit a moment. He knew by the serious expression I bore that something was up, so he skipped his usual warm and humorous greeting and sat right down. He was wearing his familiar baggy Bermuda shorts and T-shirt, a bit sweaty from just having spent awhile weeding the gardens; in fact, I could faintly smell the grass and sweat mixture. When he heard the news, his face became pained and he sat bolt upright as if struck from behind. "Oh my God, Bob. I'm so sorry. Tell me the details."

I then filled him in on the good and bad possibilities, and my resolve to see it through. I told him that Mom, Marcus, and Paul now knew and that I was about to call Polly. He, too, asked what I needed.

"Just caring at this point, Zak. We don't know yet how bad this news will be."

"That goes without saying. We're all with you."

All six foot two of him bent over and gave me a hug, which of course touched me so that I welled up in my chest and throat. I even wept a bit.

Within two days, he had given me Lance Armstrong's book, *It's Not About the Bike*. Armstrong's struggle with cancer and its treatments had been far more arduous than what I was in for, I hoped; nonetheless, his story was of faith, hope, and love as well as guts and fearless determination. Literally it meant "Never say die." I needed heroes and here was one.

One more to go tonight.

I went back upstairs to call Polly, a loving person who is sensitive and very psychologically minded. She was a talented writer and had recently compiled a book on prostate cancer for her advertising firm in New Jersey. I would find it to be well written and informative. Could this have been more than mere coincidence? I mused.

That evening, as I informed Polly, I could feel her heartache over the phone. "Oh, Bob, how awful. My heart goes out to you. And to Mom. I wish I were there with you to help."

"Just being you helps, Polly. I'm already finding love all around me. Be there for Mom, too."

"Of course I will. But you're the one who needs the most right now."

"Yes, I guess that's true, Polly, especially if my workup

is bad news. Let's pray that it won't be."

After more heartfelt exchanges, she ended with "I love you."

I was awash in blessings, but I shouldn't have been surprised. All four, in their own ways, had been devoted, loyal people who always showed me only respect and caring. I guess I was taken aback because I'd never strayed so far from the role of Big Daddy. I'd grown up with the idea of the father being the achiever, the breadwinner, the role model, and the problem solver. Also, I'd survived the silences at my childhood home by filling in the blanks and by asking for little. The resulting self-contained position evolved naturally.

I'd always espoused gender equality and had conscientiously tried to be nonsexist, but at some level I obviously had bought into the bionic "I can take care of myself" thing. In fact, as I would soon realize in the midst of the cancer fallout, the issue was not so much about gender as it was about my own developmental mythology. In other words, it was about my childhood idea that I was a star, a good boy who took care of others and achieved—and who expected to do it all by himself. And to boot, if I were really good and prayed hard, I just might get that pony in the backyard in the morning. I hadn't learned much about the other direction, of asking for and taking in help or comfort. I just gave it.

Despite myself, then, my family was now involved—not just informed, but dialed in. I was pleased that I had opened up to allow that. Their support quickly started to make a difference. The journey ahead didn't look as lonely.

Strengthened by their love and goodwill, I steeled my resolve to do the energy-demanding introspection required for maximal awareness and grounding. I knew full well that empowerment derived from both. I would start by refreshing my memory about my life story, for better and worse. I would meditate on my origins, on my family development, and see firsthand what had been and what would continue to be important parts of my crisis response. I was on a roll, so I headed toward the French doors that lead out to the deck. That quiet lovely spot overlooking the lagoon would suit me just fine.

Chapter 6

Connecting with Mom and Dad

Self-made doctor and intuitive gentle soul. Both sides of me told me that the world was my oyster, that my dreams would come true. How long did it take that little Star to grow up?

O n that evening after the bomb hit, after I had called the kids, I went outside on the center deck overlooking the lagoon, looking for some solitude. How I wished for a glass of wine—forbidden on my alkaline diet. I was tempted to suspend the alkaline diet that I'd been observing for six months. Yes, I'd lost a bunch of weight and felt smugly fit because all I consumed was veggies and some fruit. In fact, often I would imitate Bugs Bunny and tell Susan about how tasty the weeds looked—I even threatened to cut the grass by eating it. The monotony was getting to me.

I remembered the time Susan served me up one of her

famous "magic moments," complete with candlelight and promises of a surprise feast. My saliva quickened in anticipation of a nice filet, maybe a grilled grouper. In she marched, dramatically carrying the covered platter out in front of her as if bearing a gift for a prince. With a flourish and a twinkle in her eye, she placed the platter before me and removed the top.

The imp! I burst into guffaws at her artful presentation of pine twigs, palm fronds, weeds, and grass cuttings, all arranged symmetrically and topped off with peat moss. I thought I would gag from the laughter. So did she. Ever since then, the mere recollection of that moment has started me laughing out loud. We got a lot of mileage out of it for months, and it sure made the alkaline diet go down easier.

Although now I thought I deserved a break, I decided not to further blow all my sacrifice at this crucial time. After all, I'd just had champagne with Susan at our crisis summit. She readily understood, so she poured me a glass of sparkling water and carried it out to the deck for me. "Knock yourself out," she quipped.

"Thanks, pal, but I need to think."

"Just kidding," she replied in mock protest, gave me a kiss, and went back inside.

I collapsed backwards into a thick-cushioned deck chair and looked up at the sky, glistening with a gazillion stars. The three-quarter moon lit up the decks, lagoon, and bordering foliage. By now the air was a bit breezy, but still August warm. I stretched my legs out in front of me and deeply inhaled as I threw my arms overhead. The tension release settled my teeming mind.

The mere thought of more reflection brought sighs and snorts of reluctance. I'd had about enough for one day. But my comeuppance on the beach had impressed me, to say the least. I hadn't expected to discover such an immature naiveté underneath my fancy education and psychiatric expertise. What a rude awakening to the trumping power of childhood mythology like the one I'd been steeped in by my adoring parents, namely that I would win, that I would get what I wanted and what was my due, and that I would be charmed along the way.

Imagine such nonsense? You, a well-known shrink with that kind of notion under the surface? You've taught how many thousands of patients about the realities of life? You shouldn't even call it innocence. Just call it f...ed up.

But there I was on the beach earlier that day, a supposedly grown man feeling shattered and outraged. I went with the flow, knowing that the only way to get to the truth was honest exposure. So up came the tantrum into full embarrassing consciousness. My question since then has been whether what I felt is what anyone would feel at such disastrous news or whether I was, after all, in some aspects immature.

Had some of my endurance and self-confidence through fifty years been based on a boy's false bravado? Had my parents adored me so much that they unwittingly conveyed a message of my being charmed? As a boy, could I have misinterpreted their sense that I could accomplish whatever I set my mind to?

It was embarrassing to even ask such questions. Before that day's confrontation with cancer during my walk on the beach, I would have thought that I'd answered these kinds of questions in my own psychoanalysis, in my years of introspection, and especially through the thousands of patients sharing their crises. But I was so taken aback by my dismay and my tantrum that I needed to revisit the issue, so I resigned myself to yet another piece of introspective work right then and there.

I've always known that I was expected to excel, but had

either Mom or Dad actually said or implied that, as a good boy who was doing the right things, I would be immune to the dangers that beset ordinary people? Had they ever spoken about me or the rest of the world in such a way? Or had I elaborated that myth in my child's mind? I sure hoped for the latter. I just had to answer the question.

I decided to put in another fifteen minutes or so before calling it quits for the day. In a way that I had practiced for years, I closed my eyes and took long, slow, deep breaths and shifted into the zone. This time the meditation was to connect with my mother and father, now dead three and twenty years, respectively. No, I've never hallucinated or projected my astral body. No such gifts. But with deeply focused meditation, I have been able to get some sense of to-and-fro communication with them and some other important departed souls. Some would call me nuts, but such has given me comfort and grounding for many years.

How could that response have happened, Bob? Had you really harbored some preposterous assumption of a free pass? Did you not think that you, like everyone, would be faced with traumas? All you had to do was think of everyone else—family, friends, and patients—to remind yourself that all souls live with their hells and their demons. How could you have been caught so off guard? Or were you merely seeing the normal denial that allows everyone to carry on despite life's fragility and craziness?

Earlier that day I reluctantly had faced the Great Mystery and begrudgingly had to acknowledge that I had only so much to say about how my life went. In short, like it or not, I'd learned fast about the Serenity Prayer's wisdom of asking for help with the plausible, not with the fanciful. And fairness or reciprocity had nothing to do with how much hassle or shit anyone got in life. The dosage of heartache has never been, nor would it ever be, about reward or punishment or about control, except of myself.

Hell, I'd taught that for years. But now it's me on the line, and I have to know how much childishness I carry down inside.

I swallowed with an audible gulp and proceeded. The rare miracle notwithstanding, praying for specifics had never worked for me or for anyone. I'd attended to many suffering souls praying fervently for a cure for their cancer or resolution for their child's illness. The religious ones went to church regularly, dropped to their knees, and beseeched God for an outcome. No dice. In fact, the only people I'd known who had found some equanimity with their plight had been those asking for courage and strength, love, and peace. So, however reluctantly, I began to give up on the magical thinking and started to ask for help in doing the best that I could do. That evening I wanted to reflect on that for sure, but I also wanted to hang out with Mom and Dad to pull together some threads of my life.

******

New Haven, Connecticut, 1952, my big front lawn. Dad threw me a long fly ball to my right, the entire length of our front lawn. I was in my last year of Little League and was learning baseball and its lessons from my father. I chugged after it as fast as I could, arriving too late by a second or so—I wasn't exactly a speed demon. "You should've had it," he bellowed. That's what he always said when I didn't quite accomplish something or live up to his expectation. He never shamed or criticized. It's just that I should've had it. If I brought home an A−, he would ask matter-of-factly, "What happened to the A?" He wasn't being mean; he was just asking for the obvious. I chucked the ball back with my strong arm, lofting it a bit over his head so that I could

61

chide him the same way.

Even back then I loved banter. I smiled.

Those occasions of playing catch at the end of the day were relished as rare moments. Dad was a hardworking cardiologist, often arriving home exhausted and with no inclination to play. He just wanted his recliner and a few scotches. Nonetheless, he did make the time some evenings.

But there were other special occasions, like when he took me on rounds with him on Sunday mornings to Saint Raphael's Hospital. I would wait in the doctors' lounge where friendly doctors, coming and going, would greet me warmly and say nice things about Dad. "So you're Joe's son. Your dad's a heckuva doctor, you know. He took care of my aunt when she had a heart attack. He figured it out when the others couldn't. He doesn't miss much." And others, obviously his friends, said additional things about his astuteness, thoroughness, conscientiousness, and hard work. "Do you know that your old man never uses the stairs?" Then Dad would bounce in and trade repartee with his peers. He beamed and stuck out his chest when they said nice things about me to him, including my school grades and my personality. "Smart kid, Joe. Good-looking, too...must have gotten that from his mother." We all chuckled. I relished those visits to the doctors' lounge and felt warmed all over to be part of the fraternity.

******

The other times that showed me a happy father came at Yale Bowl. Saturday afternoons were for Dad and me. We saw all the Ivies play. I collected felt pennants for every school until I had them all: a crimson one for Harvard, blue for Yale, orange and black for Princeton, green for

Dartmouth, brown for Brown, light blue for Columbia, red for Cornell, and maroon for Penn. They announced my future world from their positions on our den walls at home. Of course, Dad insisted that we buy them at half price after the game.

You gotta be at least a little hungry.

Our seats were on the fifty-yard line, halfway up. Season's tickets. Big shot seats. We cheered and shouted, laughed and sang the Yale songs with the marching band. Our favorites were "Boola Boola" and "March, March on Down the Field." These were the few occasions of hearing my father, himself a Yale graduate, sing, laugh, and display unbridled enthusiasm and competitive fire. He had a fine baritone voice, and it thrilled me to hear him. He also took every penalty as a chance to comment about sportsmanship, and we applauded every injured player leaving the field, no matter the team. I learned a lot about character, passion, never-say-die attitude, and loyalty under the guidance of my hero as we sat together on the weathered wooden benches.

Right in the midst of a crucial drive inside the twenty, with all of us fifty thousand delirious spectators carrying the team with our combined cheers, a loud crackle cut through the din to jolt everyone. It came from some big place, much bigger than Yale Bowl. "Doctor Mignone," the public address system boomed in everyone's ear, "please call the hospital. Doctor Mignone, please call Yale New Haven Hospital." Well, I nearly burst with pride. God's voice was calling my father, trumping the entire spectacle. Wow. Someday I would be that important, I vowed.

Even that evening in Siesta Key reverie, my tears welled up. They always did at that memory. Of course the teams played on, but I thereafter remained aglow and resolved about my life path.

Other memories of my father were more complex—and not happy. The clink, clink of ice cubes in the glass and the glug, glug of the scotch bottle heralded Dad's usual evening drinks to "unwind." It was downhill from there as he absorbed himself in recorded music and the liquor's fog.

He sat in the same armchair every evening, and after two stiff ones, he always asked me to do the pouring and serving. "Son, would you do a service for your country?" Even at the time, the request sounded corny—drunk corny. And despite being just a kid, I had a vague sense that there was something wrong with the routine, especially in such sharp contrast to the lively man I had come to know at Yale Bowl and at the doctors' lounge. But I was, as always, a "good boy" and did what I was told. So it was out to the kitchen, open the cabinet door, and take out the half-gallon bottle to refill his glass, refreshed with more ice. I performed that service for several years despite vague misgivings. When I was in my mid-teens, my collusion was obvious to me and I stopped, offering some face-saving comment about his already seeming sleepy.

Mother always was delighted to see me return home, and I always liked greeting her. She was so classy and well-mannered, but not stiff. She was reserved and sensitive but welcomed conversation. Sadly, she was the brunt of ill-considered jibes by my father about her being an intuitive, an adept. She was intensely interested in metaphysics, had a friend who channeled, and spent a lot of time on the phone with her doing just that. My father thought it was nonsense. She kept her large library of metaphysical books tucked away in her side of their walk-in closet because in our house only Dad's values and interests had an unquestioned place.

As I sat there on the deck meditating on such memories, sadness and regret washed over fondness. I shook my head and reminded myself that all that early craziness had been just part of my journey. Maybe Dad had married her before he knew of her passion for the metaphysical, or perhaps he was enthralled by her beauty and the fact that she was a WASP art teacher and daughter of a physician from Fall River, Massachusetts. After all, he was born on a kitchen table in a poor hardworking Italian neighborhood. He loved to tell that story and was proud of having risen up and gone through Yale on scholarships. Mom, however, deserved her own credit for pushing the envelope. She graduated from Rhode Island School of Design in the 1930s—not bad for a woman in those days. From photos of her as a child, teenager, and young woman, I could see that my mother had been drop-dead gorgeous. From her forties on, though, she had hidden under forty pounds of fat and a self-effacing presentation, and she had shied away from being photographed, even if the picture was restricted to her lovely face and blue eyes.

As for me, on and off—mostly on—I may have carried thirty unwanted pounds, but I'm a ham and light up in front of any kind of camera or audience. Go figure.

My blue eyes and long eyelashes, by the way, were sources of endless compliments throughout my childhood: "Bobby, you have such blue eyes and long lashes, just like your mother." I liked that.

My mother took my father in stride, at least as far as I could tell at the time. She was too much of a Victorian lady to argue or defend herself; besides, she must have known better than to attempt meaningful conversation with a husband already losing himself in his third or fourth scotch. Before the first one, though, at dinner he indulged first Mom and then my sister, Mary, with the best cuts of meat, calling them "choice morsels." He genuinely loved making the gesture.

65

Mom would attempt to tell me about my aura, but she quickly read my loyal skepticism formed in my "alliance" with Dad and backed off into what must have been a lonely place. All she could say time and time again was, "When you're ready, you'll find many truths. You're an old soul. You'll grow up to expand your thinking. Then we can talk if you like." I didn't quite know what she was talking about, but she said it so gently and so sincerely that I loved her for it anyway. I parked those nice moments in their special place. Sadly, I missed the chance. She passed into Alzheimer's in the mid-1980s and finally left her body fifteen years later.

In my reverie, I continued my dialogue with my father.

So, Dad, what happened to the guy full of life at the hospital or football games? Why did you become an evening drunk and leave us by seven o'clock? You had it all going in your practice—reputation, pride in your work, good income. I was so proud of you except when you ridiculed Mom or took out some irritation on Uncle Fred. I recall several times walking him out to his car after a visit with you that had turned sour over some nonsense. Uncle Fred was a doll and didn't deserve your snide remarks, booze or no booze.

Besides "You should've had it," there was your other favorite, "You gotta be at least a little hungry." Even at twelve, I sensed that it meant motivation through deprivation. I also took you literally and began my lifetime struggle with weight. Remember you calling me "Chub Chub"? You may have meant it affectionately, but it stung. It has only been as an adult that I've realized you were probably referring to motivation to do one's best, never give up, and never be self-satisfied. That would give you the benefit of the doubt, because at the time I read it more as bearing the burden of never quite getting the carrot. In fact,

Dad, that's why I came to refer to you privately as "the mule," especially when there were no more wondrous moments at games and doctors' lounges.

In fact, to be painfully honest, I've continued to carry some disappointment about those issues through the years. That certainly doesn't cancel my admiration and love for your wonderful gifts and devotion to me. But it does reflect my sense of your having blown it, mostly for yourself. When you started to drink heavily, you changed. In my teen years, you essentially left me—and Mom and Mary, too. At that time, no doubt, I threw out the baby with the bath water. I felt let down. But now I know enough to realize that I didn't know what was going on inside you. I had no way to understand your sadness and caving in on yourself—still don't. So these days I can only express my empathy for you. You must have been in a lot of pain. Since being dealt this cancer situation, I've been all about compassion and forgiveness. Besides, who am I to throw stones? I've had my own "Should've known better thans."

Mom, how did you put up with all that? By my early teens, I spent all my time with friends, away from what I used to call "the morgue." Praise bicycles and cars. Remember my 1950 Ford coupe at sixteen years old, used mostly to get back and forth to school? It also delivered me into my world of sports, friends, sex, and studies. I was all over the New Haven area. You must have been terribly lonely. And to boot, I was too naïve and caught up in being an all-star son that I no doubt was insensitive to you. I'm truly sorry.

******

Then to September 1957 for a meeting of my parents, me, and the headmaster of the private day school I had attended for four years. The head man had called it to mark the culmination of my various achievements by explicitly stating the obvious to both my parents, especially my father. The real reason was no doubt to allow my parents and him a self-congratulatory glow. I, however, took it as no big thing, because all along the way I had read the report cards and comments. I had been football captain, fencing captain, editor of the school paper, member of the choir, and member of the barbershop/preppy singing group. I had won the Harvard Book Prize for outstanding junior classman and was slated for magna cum laude if I didn't screw up senior math. Classmates voted me most popular and most likely to succeed, and I was chairman of this and that.

Well, well. Weren't you something? You only had your eyes opened when you went off to college with a thousand big shots. Then how you scrambled for your identity. So much for adolescent confidence.

All had fallen into place in high school. I never stayed up and crammed. I did my workouts and studying as part of regular life in which outcomes just happened as if they were supposed to. So far as I knew, no one ever accused me of being conceited. I was just who I was and it worked, just like my parents expected. So this meeting to review college prospects was no big deal. From discussions with my teachers and class advisor, I already had figured that I probably had my pick, though I never gloated about it. It was simply the order of things. There wasn't anything to brag about because I was just being myself.

"Doctor and Mrs. Mignone, welcome to what will be a most pleasant discussion," said the headmaster. "You've known all along that Bob has been our model all-round student. My comments in all his report cards have been telling you right along how well his teachers have regarded him and how I did as well. So I'm sure it's no surprise to you to hear that Bob can pick any college or university he wants. "

My father could hardly contain himself, with a broad smile and facial flushing. My mother gracefully nodded and expressed some WASPy understated comment like, "Yes, thank you, sir. We are proud of Bob and grateful to you and your school."

I nodded nonchalantly. It was not that I felt smug; I just didn't dwell on my successes. Besides, I had already discussed this with the headmaster and with other faculty. But nevertheless I was pleased for my parents—after all, it had been their financial support and vote of confidence that had made all this possible. I had thanked them many times already, but I felt gratitude again that day.

I'd decided that I wanted to stay in New England but wanted away from New Haven. I wanted a new experience. Even at that time I realized that Boston would be a bit threatening for an insulated preppy who had grown up in a fish bowl. I thought I probably wasn't ready for even temporary anonymity, despite longing to experience both Boston and Harvard. So I bargained with myself that since Amherst College was reputed to be just as good, Amherst it was.

"What do you think, Bob?" asked the headmaster. "Knowing you, you've given it much thought."

I explained my thinking, and he agreed that it was a good choice and that I could look to early admission in the fall.

"Thank you, sir," I replied.

So, Dad, I made you proud. Your mule birthed a thoroughbred. But the price I paid in the all boys' preparatory day school was insulation from much of the real social world. I'd spent no time with women, except for

69

*weekend parties with other preppies in New Haven. While I
was polite, outgoing, and likeable, I was living in a bubble.
I only knew about high school life vicariously through
movies and television, especially "American Bandstand."
All I really knew how to do was live and excel in a rarified
world of males destined to make their marks.*

*Of course, it turned out that when I arrived at Amherst,
I found everyone to be an all-star. No more small pond.
Whatever I could do, someone did it much better, except for
one thing—people skills. That would turn out to be my forte
and the basis for my personal and professional identity. But
as for the usual academic and athletic criteria, for the first
time I was competing in a field of various geniuses, poets,
and all-star athletes. What an unsettling eye-opener.
Nevertheless, I was grateful to you both for launching me
onto that level. Back then I even felt smug about it
sometimes as I basked in the company of future scientists
and corporate leaders.*

*Dad, that sure was the path you had in mind, and
indeed it was first class. And Mom, bless your heart, you
were just happy for me. My achievements meant only that I
was fulfilling myself, at least the part that you could see.
You always loved me, fat or fit, A's or A-'s, or whatever.
Even back when I sat with you in that headmaster's
meeting hearing of my accomplishments, I was somewhat
aware that there was a whole side of me going
unrecognized. I knew that it had to do with my likeability
and my ready ability to understand people, the fact that
peers always seemed to gravitate to me with their
problems. I could always be expected to provide the
"mature" word and do the right thing when others were
being mischievous or irresponsible—and to do so without
incurring more than affectionate teasing. After all, those
same guys voted me in. I used to tell you about that side of*

myself, and you would smile and say you understood. I thanked you then, but not to the extent that I did later on and to this day. So thanks, Mom.

One more thing, both of you. What was up with my sister, Mary? I know that as the older brother and a male in the '50s, I was expected to achieve more, and I did. I know you loved her as much as me, so I've been at a loss as to why we never became close. Was I a self-absorbed jerk? I don't remember being mean to her, unless you consider ignoring her and going my own way a form of cruelty. I realize many siblings do that in their early years, but some end up being dear friends. Take Marcus and Paul, for example. They fought like hell, but now they're buddies. But as for Mary and me, not so. I'm so sad that there has been such a thin thread holding us ever since our teens. For me, the miles between us have reflected our emotional distance. I certainly have felt no animosity, and I hope she hasn't. But was I too overshadowing? Should I have done more with her? I've been in the dark about this, but I've needed to honor the problem by openly acknowledging it. I've only been able to wish her the best from afar.

******

My meditation finished up with these thoughts.

So after all is said, I don't know that I recognized anything new that night. My parents' unswerving confidence in me has always stayed with me and no doubt has given me my confidence and self-reliance. That was always explicit, so it's easy to understand. But the tougher part to grasp has been how that apparently translated to a naïve sense of special justice, namely, if I were a good boy and did the right things, I would get my dreams and wouldn't be crushed. That would be fine for adolescence,

71

but not a subconscious myth that is carried on into adulthood. I can only assume that I must have been convinced in my childhood stardom that I was charmed. Otherwise, why would I have been so righteously outraged at getting cancer? I'm embarrassed at such thinking, and I would much prefer to see it as a normal human reaction. But I still need to figure that out.

Then I suddenly felt the exhaustion from the whole day. Enough thinking, feeling, reminiscing, and figuring out. The office, the beach, the drive, breaking of the news—enough was enough. Time to get some sleep. In eight hours I'd gone from being shell-shocked to gathering my resources to looking both back and forward. Not bad for one day. All the analyzing may have been bordering on obsessing, but it was helpful in starting to get a handle on my part in this disaster.

The next task was to inform my staff and colleagues, and that needed to happen the next day. Each one deserved respect and caring and immediate involvement. I'd been through my mental gymnastics earlier on the beach as I hemmed and hawed about how and when to tell Susan. It was the same answer for telling my staff and colleagues. But with them, I also had to bear in mind both of their interests—their empathy for me and their concerns for job security. I believed in those women, so I knew they would work with me, at least until I learned whether I would live or die soon. I'd had to tell Gloria at the time of the call that day; after all, it had been she who put it through. She promised to keep it to herself until I had the chance to tell the rest of my staff the next morning. She was very supportive—not to mention shaken—but handled it with her usual grace. The next day would be the one for telling the remaining staff and my colleagues.

Chapter 7
Telling My Staff and Colleagues

Stand up, one and all. My staff: Quiet heroines show up despite private heartaches. Now they would have another—fear for my life and for their jobs. Same goes for my colleagues: Character shines again.

The time had come to tell the rest of my wonderful staff. The thirty-minute drive, on day two, down to my second office gave me the chance to rehearse. I planned to play it direct and open, just as I had so far. But this situation was more complicated than that of family or friends. These nice people had both a personal and employment agenda. I expected that as soon as each one heard the word "cancer," it would frighten them about my life and also threaten the security of their jobs. Finances would be just one of their apprehensions; losing our closely knit place of work would be another.

For ten years we'd been like a big family. I hadn't

micromanaged, and I had never raised my voice, even when an appointment error would cost me. I just took the opportunity to see if there was something to learn so we wouldn't have to go through it again. I did expect excellence, but in a face-saving way.

When I arrived, Pam, our billing person, would be busy at her computer or on the phone answering patients' questions, soliciting insurance companies about late payments, and so on. Her manner was quiet, graceful, and soft-spoken. That's not to imply that she was timid—far from it. She had always been direct, but with skill.

Betsy was, to borrow an old expression, the "hostess with the mostest." She answered the phones, made most of the appointments, and greeted all who walked through the door. Always gregarious, extroverted, and upbeat, she lent a cheery air to the reception area. She would greet me that morning from her desk with a hearty "Good morning."

Gloria P. has been my office manager for nearly fifteen years here in Florida. To say that she has been my right arm only begins to make the point; I've entrusted her with everything and anything about the practice. She has been the one to smooth ruffled feathers and resolve patients' office requests or objections. Was there a continuing problem after the first try at resolution? Go to Gloria.

Linda, a secretary/receptionist in the third office, was a conscientious gentle soul who took responsibility like a mother hen. I wouldn't see her at the office for two more days, so I would call her after talking with Gloria, Betsy, and Pam. Then I would speak with her in person upon my arrival there two days later.

The support has gone both ways for all of us. By the time many years had passed, I'd seen each of my staff through various travails of life, such as personal illnesses, family matters, and other intrusions on their lives. And no one "nickled and dimed" or counted the minutes. We were a big family and stuff happened. What was more, I admired their ability to take in stride their own traumas while staying on track and attending to patients, to me and to colleagues, and to the rest of their work. And no one would know they were hurting—talk about courage and morale.

For example, one had survived a husband with cancer and simultaneously a child with a potential neurological disaster. Another's husband had gone through open-heart surgery. A third woman's husband had recently survived prostate cancer, and she herself had survived cancer several years prior. One had chronic pain, which wasn't likely to improve, and yet another carried the burden of caring for and losing aging parents. So in one way or another, they had weathered their own storms and knew firsthand the fragility of life. Yet they carried on without an external clue, real heroines of the best kind. I believed that each one would make every effort to support me and hang in as long as the ship was still afloat.

As I drove, I visualized each of the four who would be upset at my jeopardy (one—Gloria in Sarasota—already had been apprised the day before). But I also recognized the other legitimate issue: the viability of the practice itself. Of course they would be concerned about losing their jobs if the captain went down. Who wouldn't? So I knew that I had to address both issues. And how much of myself should I reveal? How much emotional candor would be appropriate? I wanted to be honest without breeching boundaries. I wouldn't worry about becoming teary as long as the overall thrust was proactive and determined.

I'd been right. They were first and foremost concerned for my life. I took each one aside and told them my diagnosis, the details of the workup, and the gist of good and bad prognoses. I reassured each one that I would stay the course even if things got rough (of course, that would be more realistic if my workup showed no metastasis). I asked that they tell me if anything significant worried them about my behavior, my appearance, my attitude, anything—especially as it related to patient care. I made clear our priority to keep quality of care undiminished.

"I welcome...no, I insist that you tell me if you see anything off, or out of the usual, about my doctoring. And if I'm hard to work with, tell me that, too. You'll do me no favors by sparing me; in fact, that would be letting me hang myself. If I can't cut it, I'll step aside."

"No problem, boss," said the funny one of the group. "Just one exception."

"Oh, what's that?"

"If you should really go out of character and clean up your desk, that gets a pass."

Already I was breathing more lightly. I had watered up several times, but banter and jokes were always part of our office culture and had saved me from blubbering. Humor has always been natural for all of us, and there it was when we really needed it.

"Oh, one more thing. Some days I'll not be quite my usual perky self. Some days I'll be tired in the afternoon, and some days I may even not come in. If so, check my home first before you call the morgue."

No one expressed their job fears at that point—in fact, it wasn't until a year later that each confessed to me the obvious. But no one left; no one even spoke of considering another job, though no doubt that was an initial possibility. We all just kept on doing what we always had done. And we were not playing the "Emperor's New Clothes" Game. This was an example of mature people rising above personal pain to serve. I couldn't have been more grateful or proud. These were real stand-up women.

I did keep them posted at each step of the workup. We all simultaneously knew what was known at any point. We used gallows humor to diffuse the dreaded "C" word.

"Good night, Doctor. See you in the morning."

"Maybe, maybe not."

My colleagues in our group included three nurse practitioners and six therapists. To a person, they were empathic in extending support, and none of them left, either. I must admit to having had serious concerns for the financial viability of the group if some had departed. That would have been understandable, since their incomes were important for their families, but they, too, stayed the course. I was relieved to hear them discuss up front their wish to stick with me unless my status really headed south. They knew my character enough to believe that if such a decline were to happen, I would have told them directly and would have insisted that they take care of their own interests. A year after the fact, several independently said as much. Thankfully, though, my high road never required testing.

I asked myself many times in those early weeks and months if I had what it would take to hold fast to my confidence as doctor and leader through the uncertainties of the workup and treatments scheduled to run through the fall and into December. If the cancer turned out to be localized, I and all my staff, not to mention my wife and kids, could breathe a bit easier. But until the facts became clear, I couldn't let down and I couldn't offer any phony reassurances to those loyal women. Whether the cancer was local or had spread, the game had to be played all the way through.

They knew that rule of life from their general and personal experiences, and it looked like they were staying with me. But did I have the staying power? Would I crack, especially if the news was bad or the side effects worse than predicted? I tried to minimize obsessing but couldn't avoid such ordinary doubts.

******

In retrospect, my way of answering was to stick with my routine—daily workouts and unbroken work attendance. Through September, October, and November of 2003, I kept up the same packed schedule from 8:00 A.M. to 5:00 P.M. Yes, I used the men's room a whole lot but laughed it off. My staff had the grace to say nothing of it. No patient complained to any of the staff that I seemed wane or preoccupied.

I didn't inform my patients. After all, they were seeking my help, not the other way around. All of us kept patient needs front and center. As long as I could fulfill my professional duties in full, there would be no problem. Immediately, I started to watch for any significant depletion or limitations apart from the bathroom trips between appointments. I detected none. In fact, my empathy and care deepened. And I was open to any feedback from patients, staff, or colleagues. All of us had agreed to the Hippocratic principle: Above all, do no harm.

"We will not let Bob undo himself or harm patients," wrote one funny nurse practitioner on a prescription stuck to the fridge in the staff lounge. I chuckled when I read it, but I sure hoped I would still find it funny in a year from then.

******

On that second and third day of my new odyssey following the diagnosis call, two dear friends needed to get a call—rather, I needed to call them. I wasn't used to asking for help from men, but these guys were special to me. Dave and DK were both long-standing friends of good heart, substance, and loyalty. I readied myself for what I knew would be heartfelt expressions of compassion and support. The mere prospect of talking with each of them set in motion formative memories, which I shared with each. That didn't surprise me, since I figured that a man facing death did that kind of review. I savored the precious memories as if they were the very building blocks of self. So I went with the flood of reminiscences before and after each of the calls.

Chapter 8

Gathering Male Support

Self-made men and rugged individualists. Smart, savvy, and psychologically minded. Solid characters. They know the value of love and humor.

It was the second night of my reeling from the cancer diagnosis. The day before, after the wake-up call, I'd shared the news with Susan and the four kids. Then just ten hours ago, I had included my staff and close colleagues. In the meantime, the crisis had caused me to jump-start introspection about what coping skills and vulnerabilities I had brought to the table. I knew that my capacity to see this crisis through to the end would depend on my strength of heart and soul, so I was already busy with meditation and reflection.

In the previous twenty-four hours, I'd thought a lot about my early years and the important images and myths that had begun in my home and had played out in high school. Then it was time to incorporate my twenties and thirties, even my forties. That's where these two important men had formative roles, especially because they had shared with me the various mini-identity crises that had led to growth spurts. That stepwise maturation process began at Amherst College and continued to climb upwards for three decades through my years in Boston.

For that matter it has never stopped.

As has usually been the case for people, inner challenges and traumas either prompted setbacks or stimulated growth. Thankfully, I responded to the stumbles with the latter. It was somehow natural for me to tackle challenges and come out for the better. In that sense, they had been dress rehearsals for my real test—bouncing back from cancer.

Excuse me, Superdoc, but lest you gloss over the hesitation to call on friends—let alone male friends—in a time of need, you'd better admit right now that you do this out of character. It's not your usual "MO" because what you're really needing now is their—God forbid you admit it—loving support.

At the risk of stereotyping, I don't think it's just me. Most men my age don't easily ask for that. Even the enlightened among us lone warriors have fewer intimates than do women. Many of us have welcomed liberation for women, but not for us manly types. Just think about how prolific the women writers have been; there are scores of books about their surviving cancer, let alone divorce and other crises. Hell, there are academic departments of women's studies.

Knock off the lecture, Bobby. You do have two dear long-standing men friends. Count yourself lucky and reach out to them. Dial the phone.

Whichever of the two answered first would start me

pushing my own envelope for once. Each had always been psychologically astute and ready to speak freely about his inner self. What a welcome addition to my life as a young man. I'd never had a brother, and my father had certainly been smart, industrious, and accomplished, but he had not been a communicator. My teenage friends had been fun, but I hadn't reached a level of maturity for serious reflection until going away to college. That was when Dave and I became dear friends. Together we began to share the youthful machinations of finding internal freedom and acceptance. We independently shared the universal search for "Who am I?" and "What am I here for?" In my thirties and forties, I shared my inner journey with DK.

I admired both men for some similar and some different reasons. Each validated and encouraged certain of my traits and gifts that had caused me some private discomfort, namely, my intuitive and psychologically minded side. Also, I borrowed from the gifts of each, as young men and women do in their formative years. Now, when my life was on the line, all the very best in me had to come to the fore and all the very worst had to get gone—real gone.

So I welcomed the chance to immerse myself in reminiscences about those days, with particular reference to the formative contributions of these two men. They were part of my arsenal in taking on the Reaper. Their loving regard for me and their own strong attributes had become incorporated into my very fabric.

Partly because of them, my fiber became strong. I hope it'll be strong enough.

More specifically, I admired their strength of character, industriousness, astuteness, and openness to communication. Each had risen to his best possible self, climbing on no one's shoulders. They got there through honest hard work and serious thought.

Dave, for example, worked through college at a time when he was a charismatic student athlete and campus leader. He went on to become a physician and went into health administration at an international level.

DK was a lawyer, antique collector/dealer, and entrepreneur until he tired of the law and went with his boyhood passion—cars. He became a "gear-head," started his own garage for restoration of exotic cars, and built the enterprise into a world-class shop with near-exclusive expertise. He has always been a self-made piece of work.

Both were, and continue to be, true stars inside and out. They both embodied the combination of external accomplishments and recognition, and internal peace—the charismatic world leader and the rugged individualist—and both were loving men. Parts of each have lived in me and played important roles in my bouncing back from life's stumbles: That would surely be the case going forward with my handling cancer too. Also, all through the years, their connection with me has been part of the juice that I've needed to keep rising above the waves. As I noted to myself many times, that can be hard to come by, man-to-man.

It turned out that I reached Dave first. "G.B., my brother (I still called him Golden Boy from our college days), this is me from the sunshine of Sarasota." I went on to directly tell him the facts of the matter, feeling as safe as I could imagine one could feel. There was something special about the way our fraternal bond resonated with a male disease—especially one that hit us right in the jewels. He was as empathetic as I knew he would be. He asked all the appropriate questions about both the medical and personal aspects. I was happy to answer, especially about how I was coping in the immediate crisis. I reassured him that after the initial impact, I had settled in with positive resolve to see it through.

"Don't get me wrong, though. I've been scared shitless ever since the news dropped on me the other day. It's just that I'm not lying down."

"I wouldn't expect that you would, my friend. Just don't do your Superdoc thing. Ask for help. Are you letting Susan love on you?"

There was a guy who wanted to hear about my fears and sadness, about Susan's reactions and those of the kids. I easily shared, like old times.

"Thanks, my friend. I'll kick ass and keep you posted."

"You do that, hot shot. Just be real. You have people who love you."

"I know, Dave. Just kidding. Thanks again. I'll do what I need to here."

******

I hung up, and still holding the receiver, I reflected on some vignettes of those Amherst years. One of the strongest derived from the delayed adolescent identity crisis I experienced as I entered college.

I'd been a big fish and then I was a guppy. Every one around me appeared to be a star of some kind or another. So who was I? What made me special or unique? Dave and I often pondered out loud about the search for ourselves.

Since the Reaper came knocking a few days ago, I've sure as hell had to know who I am, where I'm going, and what's going to get me there. My morale depends on that, and morale will determine my staying power.

All the more reason to immerse myself in memories and reflection. These were the components of my foundation from which I would take on the cancer.

******

One evening at Amherst, sometime in the winter of 1961, Dave and I were chatting and I reflected out loud, "This place is filled with smart guys who do a lot of things well. Hell, they're all stars. Any of 'em could be an athlete, a mathematician, and a clarinetist, all at once. They're a bunch of freaky Renaissance combinations."

"Yes, Robert, my man, this is the big time. Look at you: jock, singer, resident spook, leader, and class asshole."

"Up yours, Golden Boy, you dumb jock, blonde imported hayseed of a quarterback. You walk around this place and everyone smiles and says hello, even guys whose names you can't remember because you're so dumb. Thank God they don't have to endure your dorky hick jokes."

By that time we were both holding our sides in peals of guffaws.

I've always teased and joked with those I love.

******

The most beneficial upshot of my four years of college was mostly internal. I ended up resolving the question of my individuality by basing it on my people skills, intuition, and psychological mindedness. I got positive feedback about leadership skills and likeability all four years. As I'd come to recognize since the cancer crisis began two days before, that bedrock self-concept would be crucial to my taking on the cancer because after all is said and done, the recovery experience would largely be an inner journey of holding fast to my identity and morale.

So whatever kind of shit hit the fan, I would always have myself to fall back on and my inner strength to let me reach out to love. And besides, lifesaving laughs were only possible from a solid sense of self.

******

The next evening I reached DK. Leading up to the call, I paused to fondly remember his image. He was a slim, wiry man who had always marched to his own drummer. He was the very model of creating his own manhood without much external support because his interests were not necessarily what his family considered mainstream. For them, he had become a lawyer and had built a successful practice until his passion for cars pulled him away. He developed a garage that eventually turned out to be world-class. He also loved antique collectibles of all kinds, including houses; in fact, it was in one of his old Salem houses that I set up my practice in the early '70s. As I have said, he was one of a kind.

For many years in the 1980s, we would meet in the early mornings and walk around Salem. The companionship was warming and the conversation most enlightening. DK was very astute and verbal about what made people tick. He and I spoke at length about our life stories, especially the challenges to overcome. We shared a commitment to personal growth through developing self-awareness and pushing the envelope.

He, like Dave, went where my father never could go—to talk about the emotional side of life. So I had validation about my intuitive gifts. This was not psychobabble; he was on the money to the point where I often thought he could have been a shrink rather than a car nut or a lawyer. He was another male with whom I could identify and derive inner warmth. Like Dave, he was part of my building blocks. He too had risen above life's challenges, and I had shared some with him. I was about to ask him to share in my biggest one. Time to dial...

"DK (I didn't have to identify myself since only I called him that—I've always had nicknames for my loved ones), I have some potentially bad news, my friend. Yes, you'd better sit down. And take off that silly cowboy hat you're probably wearing. I have prostate cancer."

I went on to spell out the details. As always, he was endlessly curious about every one. He asked more detailed questions than anyone to date because that was his way, endlessly inquisitive, but that evening his inquiries were heartfelt. He expressed the loving best wishes that I expected from a man as solid as he was. He asked to be kept abreast of developments.

"Of course I will, my friend. Hopefully I'll be riding around the North Shore with you next summer in one of your antiques." Then we said our good-byes and made promises to stay in touch.

As I hung up, it occurred to me that DK's importance to my inner acceptance went even beyond his modeling of fierce independence and his acceptance of whoever I was. He also had an incredibly open mind about things like alternative medicine long before it became mainstream. He even asked me to perform acupuncture on his back.

He was and has remained another strong male figure who is both manly and sensitive—and can laugh about it. No wonder I called on him during my crisis.

******

Especially since I'd never had a brother or a communicative father, Dave and DK had been important males in my life. Our shared experiences, especially those that asked me to resolve a dilemma in order to go forward, had been part of my shaping. They might have been mini

88

wake-up calls or just challenges, but my response to each one further built my resilience and confidence.

It was like going full tilt in sports, knowing I might be unexpectedly injured at any time, but if I were, I would get back in the game having learned more about both myself and the game.

Needless to say, Bud, this cancer is the game of your life.

******

I took the time that evening in the glow of the warm phone conversation to reflect more. I sat back in my desk chair in my den from which I had made the call to DK and allowed myself to drift off. One vivid memory of starting medical school came to mind as a cementing of my calling to medicine and my alliance with that part of my father, the physician.

Jump forward to Duke Medical School, first-year anatomy class. The laboratory odor of preserving chemicals burned my nostrils. My stomach was queasy, and my eyes were heavy. All of us fledgling med students, in spanking new starched white lab coats and aliens in a new world, gathered in the gross anatomy lab containing a dozen corpses laid out supine on operating tables. Each was draped with a hospital sheet so all we could see was the poking up of a nose, the mounds where breasts probably lay, a belly protuberance, and bare feet sticking out at the end. We assembled for the introductory remarks from the professor. I felt at once like I was in a chapel, a funeral home, and a laboratory. I shuddered at the thought of unveiling one of those bodies so as to begin carving it up, even in the name of science.

The professor was somber yet certainly not morbid.

"This is a sacred place in which you must hold reverence. We are grateful to the spirits of these departed who have offered their bodies for your learning. Your conduct in this laboratory must at all times reflect your appreciation by, among other things, quiet comportment and serious intention. You socialize and blow off steam outside of here. Think of this as being in church."

Tension inside me eased up a bit, but I still dreaded the imminent unveiling.

"Before you unveil your cadaver, consider whether or not you are prepared to offer your own body in return at the time of your death. If you would not be willing to do so for future medical students, perhaps you should think again before embarking on this path."

I guessed I could do that someday. The whole experience sure was serious and bigger than life.

Welcome to medicine.

******

Then fast-forward a year to second-year med school where I faced a mini-crisis of professional identity in my physical diagnosis course. Just as I was beginning to be pleased with my honors-level classroom performances, I started my first course in physical examination.

What a thrill!

I'd finally arrived at the moment of being a doctor with real live patients to interview and examine on the floors. Yes, I had gotten A's in the classroom and laboratory basic sciences, but now for doctoring—that was where I would really shine. That was my destiny, the second generation of doctors (unless I counted my maternal grandfather, which would make it the third). Anyway, I was promulgating the best of the Mignone mythology of excellence, persistence, and morality in service.

Our long-awaited physical diagnosis practicum was scheduled for one of the internal medicine wards at the Duke VA Hospital. Four classmates and I were to rendezvous at a given hour and meet with the professor to set the timetable for the examinations and follow-up group discussion. Then we were to disperse to assigned patients. I arrived thirty minutes early, barely restraining my enthusiasm. My heart rate rose to over 100 beats per minute. Hell, I was just plain high. In my right hand, I clutched the pharmaceutical company–donated shiny black leather bag filled with stethoscope, blood pressure cuff, ear and eye lights, reflex hammer, and such. I proudly wore my white lab coat, the uniform for all doctors in the hospital. Mine didn't say M.D. on the name patch yet, but I was in the ball game.

"Gentlemen, you have forty-five minutes to get a history and perform a physical exam on the patient whose name you see beside yours on this list. Enjoy your first experience at live medicine. We'll meet in the conference room to discuss your findings. We may visit one or two of your patients and ask you to present at the bedside. There's no better way to learn to swim than to get in the water. Good luck."

All five of us in our study group parted and headed down the hallway looking for the room housing our assigned patients. I nearly skipped down the hall but managed to refrain in the name of professional composure. At some level, I knew that I must have looked like a gawky novice, but on that day I saved my confidence by dragging up an image of my father's famous bedside manner.

All I was given was a room number and the man's name. I paused at the doorway and checked the number and name tag on the door to make sure I was in the right place.

Yup. This is The Show.

My heart flip-flopped as I was about to enter my new world. I could almost hear the roar of the crowd and a faint strain of "Boola Boola."

I took a deep breath, exhaled, straightened my back, and strode in with a gait that I hoped conveyed both self-assurance and respectful manners. Not too eager, but definitely pleased to be there to help.

"Good afternoon, Mr. Johnson. I'm Robert Mignone, a third-year medical student. I would like to ask you about your health history and perform a physical examination if you are still agreeable with that. If this becomes too tiring or distressing, just say the word and we'll stop."

He lay quietly on his back, sheets up to his chest and unperturbed by my entrance, and he appeared to be looking at something on the ceiling. He didn't answer, but he also didn't object, so I proceeded to his bedside. "What brought you into the hospital at this time, sir?" He wasn't responding to my questions.

"That's OK, sir. If it's too difficult to talk right now, we'll skip that part. But I would like to proceed with an exam, OK?" When he didn't object, I took out my stethoscope and placed it in different positions over his heart, searching in vain for a beat. Then I heard one. But was that the beating of my own pulse in my ears against the ear pieces of the stethoscope?

Oh my, this is harder than I thought it would be. He has a barrel chest, so maybe that's why his heart and breath sounds are so distant or even inaudible.

Damn my stumbling. Dad is a cardiologist and reputed diagnostician. What the hell am I?

I swallowed the rising tide in my chest and shined the light in his eyes to see if he would startle. He didn't. Just big pupils that didn't shrink in the light beam.

This will not do. He's probably in a coma from some neurological catastrophe or metabolic problem. He has a curious odor that I've heard is part of liver failure.

A few more failed attempts to test his reflexes and move a limb told me to quit and go fetch the professor. This case was more complicated than one for a new medical student.

The professor and I went to the bedside. My heart sank to my shoes and my face flushed hot, and shame excoriated me in my mortification—the patient was dead, quite dead. From the professor's findings, the patient had died several minutes or so before I had arrived.

I was the stupidest, most inept, and most ridiculous excuse for a doctor that ever entered the field of medicine, let alone Duke. "Fallen star" didn't begin to capture the ignominious moment, nor would "comet crash."

I could see the headline: "Class Hotshot Blows First Physical Exam, Fails to Diagnose Death." An alternative headline in my head read: "Stricken Schmuck Sucks Wind: Couldn't Diagnose Humanity's Most Common State." Better still: "Duke Needs Real Doctors, Not Imposters."

My humbling couldn't have been more complete. My voice trembled as I offered an apology, and I felt like crying and crawling under the hospital bed. But God bless Dr. Flanagan. He was sensitive and empathic. "Don't worry, Bob. This is your first day. This kind of thing happens all the time in the beginning. I've been there myself. This is the strange new world of medicine, Bob. It'll only get better from here." I was speechless....Verbal, articulate me.... Dumbfounded.

Dr. Flanagan saved my face by telling none of my peers that I'd blown it, by converting the teaching exercise into an opportunity to see the findings of recent death. After all, we would need to know these for our future responsibilities of pronouncing death.

That was the first time my idealized expectations crashed. It was worse than the identity machinations after entering college. The importance of identifying as a physician could hardly have been greater, so the blindsided hit of my screw-up had me reeling for days. I trashed myself, prompting immediate soul-searching to come up with a more realistic and gentler self-image. I also rose to the occasion and vowed to become the best possible diagnostician. As it has turned out through the years, my physical diagnosis and history-taking skills have been crucial elements in my clinical accomplishments.

Out of that crisis resolution arose an accelerated strength of purpose and determination, attributes that eventually were to directly strengthen my response to any crisis or challenge, especially cancer. In effect, I took a possibly crushing—or at least a staggering—blow and turned it into learning.

Because of that kind of positive attitude about responding to threats and hits, I had come to know pretty much who I was, what I stood for, and how I could stay on top of my game. Of course, little did I realize until the bomb exploded just days before that I was in for the biggest test of my resilience. Before the cancer jolt, I had believed in my brains, heart, and soul, but after the cancer call I sure as hell was going to be tested. I would need every bit of my confidence going forward. Seeing this big picture of my sequential growth through building on mini-crises helped a lot to cement the pieces and strengthen that resilience.

That was why I kept reviewing and going over my life story of meeting setbacks, at times to Susan's exasperation. "Oh, Sigmund...are you still obsessing?" she called down the stairway.

"Yeah, sweetheart. But I'm almost done for tonight. I'll

be up in a few minutes. Let's watch a silly movie or something."

I wasn't quite finished with reminiscing, so I resumed revisiting my med school process of emerging from under the weight of paternal expectations into a personal commitment to psychiatry.

******

The track I created for myself in med school was traditional research academics because that was cool in medicine for an honors student hotshot, and most definitely cool for my father. And it certainly prevailed among my peers, especially the top students who essentially took one side of the Cartesian split between mind and body. In the 1960s, the buzz was all about the body. Biophysics was king, and there was a love affair with technological, "objective," science in those days; anything else was second- or third-rate. Being a thoracic surgeon or neurosurgeon was cool, and being an OB-GYN or radiologist was okay—what was ridiculed was psychiatry.

Besides revisiting my worst medical nightmare in physical diagnosis class, confronting my ultimate decision about professional direction was probably the most determinative of my Duke experience. As one of the honors students deemed capable, there I was in the midst of a culture that valued above all else becoming a research-oriented professor of internal medicine or surgery; however, my growing curiosity and natural ease with bedside medicine and the humanity of illness demanded bucking that prevailing tide, so to speak. I just couldn't get on board the academic express steaming to corporate research academia. Perhaps my mother's influence began to grow, as the psychology/medicine interface beckoned.

The first day I entered a psychiatric ward named after the famed Dr. Adolf Meyers, I was hooked. I was terrified, fascinated, and energized. I was in the place everybody feared and felt the need to detoxify or demystify by making fun of it. Names like "spooks" and "shrinks" took care of the "wackos" and the "crazies." Even the strong and the mighty in the faculty stayed away.

Admittedly, it was the psychiatric age of rudimentary treatments such as insulin shock, electric shock, and only a couple of medications, so there wasn't much to do for very ill patients. Most of my peers back then regarded psychiatry to be in the "dark ages" in comparison to the other specialties. I, however, saw it as a field bound to explode into new frontiers. Therefore, I became a target when I threw myself into psychiatric reading and clinical contact with a fervor that was much stronger than that of my peers, who just wanted a good grade.

"Why the hell is an honors student like you interested in that stuff? Have you gone crazy too? You're an A.O.A. You could do what you want!"

"Are you shitting me? A spook? That's for the guys who can't do anything else."

I was a puzzle all right, to my peers, to my teachers, and certainly to my father. He, too, couldn't fathom anything for me but being the all-star on the academic stardom track. He told me so directly, couching his skepticism as questions. Mother, however, was no doubt quite pleased in seeing me start to openly embrace my intuitive and creative side. After all, psychiatry could be as broad as I wanted it to be, interfacing neurology and internal medicine on one hand and the arts on another. I was on board.

That had been the most important step to date in my professional identity, but at a private level, it was the most openly stated acceptance of my so-called right brain side. I came out of the closet, so to speak, and openly declared my identification with the psychological aspects of medicine and of my own humanity. My inner growth accelerated through subsequent years by being able to embrace intuitive metaphysical and spiritual aspects of myself and of medicine.

As I sat in my den and saw that kind of broad picture, I was struck at how much my doctoring has always depended on—and reflected on—my person. And in that same vein, it was rapidly becoming clear that my spiritual and psychological strengths—so important in my responses to various challenges through the years—would damned well be crucial in taking on my cancer.

Robert, my man, thank your stars, or whatever, that you've had the good stuff you were given, the experiences you were presented, and the ways you took on the journey. You may have taken a knee now and then, but you never went down or at least stayed down—you got right back in the game. Now we'll see what you're really made of. Call on what you've learned and how you've coped, buddy, because you're going to need it. And you're going to need the love of your wife and children, your staff and colleagues, and your guy friends to pull this one off.

******

The final coup de grace to doubts about going with my intuitive/psychological side as a man and physician came in neurology residency. When I and my fellow residents actually held in our collective hands a human brain at autopsy and drew through it the special knife for brain cutting, I was shaken to my core. Was I going to look primarily inside physical brains and spinal cords, or was I mostly to examine emotional and spiritual aspects of people? I was compelled to move toward the psycho-spiritual side of life and of medicine but not sacrifice anything in the requisite skills of physical medicine and practical daily living.

I must have conveyed my ambivalence throughout that year because for the first time in my life, I was not invited to return to a sought-after position in academia. I didn't know whether to feel relief to be off the hook (since I had already decided not to return) or to feel chagrined at failing. The relief triumphed.

******

My ass began to ache, but I couldn't resist a couple of minutes in a more positive vein. My public declaration of who I was reached its zenith with my acceptance into the psychiatry program at Mass General Hospital, Harvard Medical School.

July 1, 1970, was my first day of work at "the Mass Jesus," as it was affectionately called. I was like a boy getting an autograph from "the Babe" himself. I was feeling starstruck and giddy as well as chomping at the bit, all at the same time. I walked up Fruit Street toward the legendary hospital as it loomed skyward like a great European cathedral. I'd landed on another planet and was about to enter the mother ship. I strode up to the huge entrance doors with all the confidence I could muster but with my exuberance bridled. I didn't know whether I felt more like a kid in a fairy tale candy store or a novitiate entering the hallowed Vatican. I'd never before experienced anything so simultaneously thrilling and humbling. I entered the cathedral lobby with its waiting room of sumptuous leather chairs. As I approached the information desk to ask for directions to my destination in the enormous complex, I was awash in nausea. I frantically made it to the men's room just in time to throw up in a toilet.

Welcome to The Show, Superdoc. I grinned as I rinsed my mouth and spat into the porcelain sink.

My tenure went well there at MGH. I loved psychiatric scholarship and clinical practice, and the exalted status of MGH no doubt helped me with my internal struggle to validate those "soft" sides of myself. To this day I wonder how I would have found peace, absent such a strong "social parent-figure." Anyway, it all came fairly naturally then and has ever since. Finally, I was home.

******

And speaking of home, how about Susan, my woman? Here I sit, downstairs from her, meditating away while she does her independent woman thing. I've been continually grateful to her for many things, not the least of which are her loving support and dependability through this cancer crisis. I know she'll stay the course.

Three days ago, the cancer bomb dropped on my head. I've been in high gear since, gathering my support, informing those who needed to know, and thinking a lot about my life story and how it pertained to the strength or weakness of my cancer response. I know enough to realize that whatever level of resilience I can muster will be a product of a lifetime of experience sustained by love and humor. Thinking hard about the formative men in the past two days had been enriching and reassuring. Indeed, I've been educated in a world of men all along, so there have been many influential male teachers, coaches, and friends.

But enough is enough for tonight.

99

"I'm on my way up, sweetheart. Be patient. After all, I may be a dead man."

As I climbed up the winding stairs to Susan, I heard her giggle in reply. It occurred to me that her birthday was coming up soon. I'd been so preoccupied that I'd forgotten. I'd always done something special for her, but this year I would make a bit more of a fuss.

Chapter 9

Susan

All the good stuff, plus beauty and humor. No task too big. Loves me and loves her family and friends. A signature laugh filled with mirth. What a woman!

O ctober 21, 2003, was Susan's birthday. I'd just started radiation treatments and was doing okay. I hadn't missed a day at the office or at the gym. My day still began at 6:00 A.M. and was full all the way until 5:00 or 6:00 P.M. To be sure, I'd been retiring an hour earlier, but a small price to pay. As Susan teased whenever I complained, "It beats the box." Her humor, love, and grounding had already started to be instrumental in my coping.

I finished setting up for a candlelight birthday dinner out on the deck overlooking the pool and the lagoon. The flickering candles offered a pleasing faint citrus fragrance; the table was set resplendent with our favorite handmade

Vietri pottery and glasses; champagne was on ice in a nearby bucket, poised for the happy birthday pop; and filets were in the fridge while the grill stood at the ready with top open and grid scrubbed. As corny as it may sound, each year I commemorated Susan's birthday in gratitude for her birth that brought her into my rebirth. This evening was the more sweet for my being alive and hoping that I would see many more.

I took a moment to sit down in one of the wicker chairs and reflect. The setting couldn't have been more magical: The candles glowed softly, casting some soft shadows beyond the furniture; some were also moon shadows, from the big bright orb shining against the galaxies of sparkle lights that paint our vast canopy out there. I had to believe in the cancer therapy I had chosen so that I would live to see many more birthdays. My chest tightened and my eyes started to fill up.

No, you're not going there. Stay in the moment, this lovely moment. Think about Suzy. She's been your partner for years and recently has come through in spades.

******

It was May 1989 at the front door of Susan's funky cottage on a lake north of Boston. We had met awhile back through mutual friends. By the time I arrived, it was 9:30 P.M. or so, too late for the local restaurants. No matter, I figured we could forgo food, or she might be able to put something together. I knocked, eager to see the pretty blonde who had reminded me of a Norwegian beauty in film. My heart rate picked up, and I was giddy with anticipation.

She opened the door and I was smitten. Her blonde hair, fine like a girl's, was up in a top knot at an askew angle.

Her sumptuous lips and mouth formed a huge welcoming smile. Her almost husky voice enhanced the warmth as she greeted me in a cheery tone. Then as I stepped toward that angel, I noticed the boxes in the entrance about the entry hall; some were packed and sealed, and some were open, half filled with books or glassware.

"Am I interrupting something here? Are you coming or going?"

"Going," she replied half apologetically. "But come in. Let's spend my last minutes here together. No, I'm kidding. But please, come in and make yourself at home—what's left of it."

We laughed, partly to relieve tension but also because she was downright funny.

Great, so now she's not only beautiful, sensual, warm, mannerly, and friendly, she's also funny. And leaving town. Terrific.

But my nature had me press on, determined that I might find a way to get to know her. We tried a couple of local restaurants that appeared open, but by late evening they were only serving beer and wine. So she suggested that we return to her place and she would cook us dinner.

Wonderful. Also a cook. We could talk uninterrupted.

By this time I was captivated by her manner, wit, and warm, earthy energy. And could she laugh, like no woman I had ever heard before. She threw back her head, in a lusty yet feminine way, and wholeheartedly giggled or bellowed or shrieked like a delighted girl. At times her laugh almost sounded musical. It was infectious.

Absolutely distinctive! This woman is a keeper. She might be on her way to California, but there are phones and planes.

So it was back to her lake house for dinner. I took a glass of wine and sat in the nearly barren living room while she set to work in the kitchen preparing dinner.

"Bob, do you like pizza?"

"Sure, who doesn't? That'll be fine, but don't go to a lot of trouble."

"Oh, don't worry, I won't. I'll bring it out in a second."

Shortly thereafter, she appeared carrying two plates with small pizzas. She was smiling, but I couldn't tell it if was whimsy, apprehension, or embarrassment. Quickly I figured it to be all three.

"They didn't quite come out the way my mother-in-law used to make them," she grimaced out of the side of her mouth. "Not quite like Pizza Regina, either," as she held my plate out for me. On it sat an untoasted English muffin topped with a slab of cold cheddar cheese and finished with a topping of a raw tomato slice. I suppressed any hint of laughter, took a small bite to investigate, and with a straight face offered the overused expression that allowed a thousand possibilities: "Interesting." Then I had nowhere to go but to ask, "What is it?"

"Pizza!" she exclaimed with put-on incredulity. "The Italian doesn't know a pizza when he sees one?"

Then I lost it and burst with laughter, nearly spitting out my sample. I rocked back into the sofa, clutching my stomach with one hand. She, too, burst into peels of guffaws and squeals of mirth. She almost dropped the plate.

"Good, right? Took a lot of pains with that one right there."

I coughed and coughed as my next round of laughs hit.

"Oh, come on. You can say it. I'll bet you never had one like that before."

This woman is a scream. Beautiful and funny? Gimmeabreak!

I started to hum out loud the refrain, "California, here I come."

"Oh, you're coming for more of these? Good taste. They're even better with California tomatoes."

Well, the rest of that evening passed on a cloud for both of us. There was no time to be cool or strategic. She was supposed to leave in a few months, so I made my intentions known, and she, hers.

"Go right ahead with your plans. You've been dreaming about sunshine for a long time. And if you want me to, I'm right behind you with plane trips and lots of phone calls. I'm coming after you until you tell me to go away."

"Oh yes, by all means, Bob, come out. And yes, we'll stay in touch by phone."

Nearly fifteen years ago, her humor broke the ice, kept the action going, and created magic out of what could have been a real downer. She helped me go forward with a courtship under circumstances that might have seemed insurmountable.

Nice start.

******

On one of our first dates soon thereafter, we talked about one another's lives, where we had been and where we wanted to go. From my wicker chair on the deck fifteen years later, I still felt a mixture of surprise and relief upon discovering early on that she hardly had listened to my insecure recitation of credentials. There I was, laying out my precious academic lineage and she could have cared less.

What a dork.

She only seemed interested in hearing about my personal life, my dealings with people. Clever person that she was, she was scoping me out as a person, a man—a potential friend and/or partner.

You're lucky she didn't hear you really go into your insecurity thing about achievements. Even with the amount you did say, you must've sounded like you were applying for a job. Real attractive, Dork.

She admitted to me much later that all she could recall, even that evening, was something about Yale and Harvard, but not the rest of the lineup. Those status labels weren't what she was interested in. She later told me, "I was listening to your voice."

I was perplexed at first. I knew she was smart because there are no funny, witty dummies. I just hadn't met a beautiful, warm woman who was primarily interested in my personal qualities, or maybe more to the point, I'd never recognized them because of my focus on my own externals. Anyhow, what she wanted to know about was my personality, my values, and my maturity. As she had made clear on our first meeting, she was only interested in a man, not a boy. The pedigree world had not been her chosen turf. For many reasons in her background, despite a very sharp mind she never went the achievement route. Instead, she was a social and interpersonal natural. She had many friends, was often the life of the party, and was always the social organizer. There's no framed diploma for that one.

Within a week, we kissed for the first time. All those songs about heaven moving and the books and movies about the first kiss foretold that moment. My knees really did buckle, my heart flip-flopped, and my head felt woozy. Her full soft lips were like velvet, the skin on her face was smooth as a baby's, and her perfume, subtle as it was, was intoxicating. Susan seemed dazed, stumbling for words, and turned to get into her car to drive home. We had each arrived with our own vehicles. I floated home to Salem. She told me the next day that she had become lost on her way back to her lake house, traveling roads that she knew as well as her driveway. We had some laughs about that one, too. I gave her a tape of Jimmie Cliff's song, "You Can Get It If You Really Want It."

I visited California several times over two months. We spoke daily on the phone and also wrote love letters. Fourteen years ago it sure looked to everyone like a foolish rush. Undaunted, we held our private covenant ceremony in the garden of a California Spanish-style B&B in which we were staying for the weekend. We exchanged rings, just the two of us.

Had it been too fast? My two sons and her son and daughter thought so, out of common sense, as did our individual friends. We understood but pressed on, knowing we had something special and serious. Time would ease their doubts.

Maybe it was just dumb luck, but Susan turned out to be just what I had needed. I've preferred to consider the connection providential. Our tastes, loving commitment, and values were very much the same. She was psychologically minded and astute, and I could tell that she had the wisdom of an old soul. And she knew how to laugh at the nonsense of life, let alone break the tension of certain heavy moments with a wisecrack. Besides that, she was delicious. And she loved me, too. We've had the same outlook about no bombast: When people behave well, there should be little need for carrying on; skillful talking should resolve the hurt or whatever. And it has.

She came along at a time when I was ready for a sea change. Her own capacity to rise above adversity through her life had impressed me as I learned about it. That same trait helped us get through a start-up that would have derailed many couples. Little did I know then that fourteen years later her resilience would be a vital part of my taking

107

on the threat to my life.

I shifted in my seat on the deck, checked that the candles were still burning, and listened for Susan's car in the drive. No sound of her approach. She must still be either at Siesta Beach or on her way home. So I shifted back to reflecting on Susan and her part in my life before and since the cancer bomb.

No wonder she's been so important in already helping me to respond constructively and positively to cancer. It hasn't been just that she loves me. She has always chosen climbing mountains over taking detours or turning back. And besides that, her old soul wisdom and intuition have allowed her to know just when I've needed to lighten up and when I've needed some slack to do my psychological-spiritual meditation thing.

******

After a year of courtship, we married. It was in August 1989, just days before our move to Florida. For the big occasion, we blew our savings by renting a white clapboard country estate with lovely flowering grounds on the north shore of Boston. It was surrounded by country gardens and was the picture of New England summer. Sprawling and spacious, it promised ample room for indoor buffet dining and dancing to complement the out-of-doors strolls. All of our families and friends were invited (by that time we had their confidence).

The morning of the grand indoor/outdoor wedding, it poured like a monsoon in the Pacific. Sheets of rain beat down so hard that one could barely see fifty feet at times. A couple of older family members cancelled out of concern for the driving. Disaster was imminent. All our wedding dreams—let alone spare money—had gone into this summer wedding extravaganza. We knew many who had bought new summer dresses and matching shoes. It was to be the real deal.

My heart was sinking, and I started to pace and wring my hands. Forecasts predicted no letup. I worried about Susan and her big day and felt terrible for her. I was also pissed about God allowing Mother Nature to spoil our day of all days. Then, with what I came to learn was her irrepressible impish nature, Susan announced that I should go up to the corner sporting goods store and purchase two snorkeling outfits.

"Are you daft? Sweetheart, we don't have time for nonsense," I said incredulously. I was sure it was just another wisecrack.

"Bob, I'm serious. Just trust me on this. Take ten minutes and run up there and get face masks, snorkels, and fins. And don't forget the fins."

"You're serious, aren't you?"

"Yes. Everyone will arrive all dressed up and will have to run through a waterfall. They'll be so furious about ruining their new shoes and hats that when they see us standing in the doorway dressed up in our wedding finery with fins, snorkels, and face masks, they'll pee their pants. So please go. And as you're cursing your own drenching on your way up the street, think of the looks on their faces when they come out from under their umbrellas."

"Brilliant! You're a piece of work. I'm off."

I chuckled all the way to and from the store.

We stood in the doorway to greet everyone as they frantically dashed from car to house through the puddles, desperately clutching their umbrellas. There we waited at the front door: I in suit and tie, she in a new formal dress, and both with the added diving gear.

As I sat on the deck awaiting Susan's arrival for her

birthday feast, I burst into uncontainable laughter at remembering the astonished looks on the faces of our guests. Immediately after their double-take, they burst into belly laughs. Some literally fell into our arms in apoplectic laughter. The buzz of the party quickly converted the mood and energy to levity and goodwill. Jokes about sloshing shoes and droopy hats just caused more raucous laughter through the early evening as tensions dissipated.

All these years later, neither of us can look at our wedding photos with a straight face. That was pure genius. And how different was that from eight weeks ago when she rescued us both from morbidity with her champagne joke? Or just a few days ago when she said, "Before you croak, could you take out the trash?"

As they say in Rhode Island, "You gottaluvit."

******

Still listening out of one ear for the crunching sound of her car tires, I continued my thoughts. Susan's importance to my life to date had been one thing, but as I faced possible death, her ability to put herself in my place and resonate with me, her astute use of well-placed humor, and her grit had already been crucial. And her natural wisdom had helped immensely in my holding to my purpose. I was sure those contributions would continue to be vital, especially over the longer haul of the upcoming side effects. In those days after the cancer crisis hit, what could have been gallows watching turned into constructive coping and even healing.

I hope I can keep up both.

There! The sound of tires on crushed shell! She was home. Now was my time to indulge her with a delicious meal and fine champagne. I would break my fast for the

110

second time this fall. We would no doubt reminisce about the past fourteen years, but I wanted to avoid any talk of cancer. I certainly didn't want to even vaguely mention the fact that this might be one of the last of her birthdays with me—we would not spoil the evening's mood. We'd talked plenty about all that for two months now, ever since the abnormal PSA had come back and the biopsy had been performed. I'd already told her what I'd read and what I'd had been told about the need to pee often and the possible pain, my impending chemical castration, and, ultimately, the seed implants. It sounded like some men had a really bad time of it. There would be no beating it to death, surely not this evening.

"Hey, birthday girl."

Part 3

Taking It On

Chapter 10

The Options

Cut it, bomb it, freeze it, burn it, starve it. No easy choices, but the atomic bomb looks like a go.

Back to the first week, after the big day. Loved ones, friends and family, and staff and colleagues now were on board. Their collective prayers and good wishes created a well of determination to get down to business. So I started what turned out to be many hours in front of the computer, both at home and at the offices. I pulled up prostate cancer and was shocked at the sheer number of references. I should have expected as much, since this is our number one male cancer behind lung cancer—and the numbers are big.

My search engine turned up surgery, oncology, radiation-oncology, and alternative medicine citations, depending on the buzzwords that I used. I poured through them until the information became repetitive. I made notes. I weighed the efficacy data, evaluated the side effects and downtime, and looked into who and what were available in the region. Needless to say, all the thinking depended on whether the cancer was localized to the capsule around the gland or whether I was riddled with it. That workup remained, but at least I learned the decision tree.

Luckily, after all the asking and reading and thinking, there were top surgeons and radiation oncologists close by. Therefore, either localized or systemic treatments, or both, were possibilities, so I could consider all options. Had I lived elsewhere, I might not have been so fortunate.

I set aside an evening with Susan to go over all this information so that I could come to a decision. I wanted to run by her all the realistic options because she would be living through all of the treatment results and side effects with me. And, obviously, she would be looking for the same thing I was—to escape death with effective treatment. So on that evening, still in the first week of post-cancer news, I gathered my notes and went upstairs to the living room to find her. This time, as I ascended the stairs, there was bounce to my step. All the work of the past several days had paid off: I was being proactive and feeling some of my old kick-ass energy. I would not allow thoughts of failure. What would be the point? All I could control was what I had been doing and what I would do.

"Sweetie, please sit with me on the sofa so I can go over all this with you. Much of the medical detail will be read out loud for my sake. I'll watch for your glazed-eye look and be brief, but for obvious reasons I must be complete."

"Don't worry about me. You just start talking. The part I have to know is what stands the best chance of cure. As for side effects, we'll live with doing whatever we have to."

"OK, fair enough. Just don't pull a fade when it's too detailed. Tell me to explain."

"Of course. Now don't you start worrying about my brain, Smart Guy. Just because I wanted to grow up to be a cigarette girl…you know, the short fluffy skirts and the net stockings and heels, and the tray of…"

"OK, OK. I'm sorry. Just let me do this."

I thought it best to start out with an explanation of the prostate's function and how it's affected by cancer. I didn't want to assume that she knew the anatomy that was demanding our attention. With some trepidation about sounding like a biology lecture, I started out, "First, let me describe the prostate itself."

"Oh, you mean that thingie somewhere up in there that does something for men?"

"Come on, sweetie, I'm serious."

"I know. I'm sorry. Just trying to lighten you up, Doctor. Please go on."

"OK. First, the prostate is a uniquely male organ—you don't have one. It's the size of a walnut and sits at the neck of the bladder."

"Thank God. At least I don't have to worry about prostate cancer. My breasts are targets enough."

"Bear with me, sweetie. I know you want bottom line without the medicalese, but I need to do it this way. And you need to hear it, despite your 'blonde' put-on. OK?"

"Sure, go ahead."

"The urethra, or urine tube, runs out through it and courses through the penis. The prostate's job is to secrete a fluid that is part of a man's semen. The other part comes from the testes. To visualize this, imagine the prostate gland as a lime and the urethra as a straw. The lime sits right next to the bladder, and the straw runs from the bladder directly through the lime and continues out through the penis. It opens at the penis head to discharge urine. This is how men empty their bladders."

"I didn't know that was how men go tinkle."

"Settle down…I realize you probably know some of this, but I'm just trying to be clear….So if the lime swells or develops a mass, the straw can be compressed and then symptoms start. If inflammation is part of the swelling, burning pain is included. If the straw is compressed too much, it collapses on itself and an obstruction happens. At that point, school's out: Get to a doctor or the ER."

"Uh, huh. And…?"

"Bear with me. Compromised urinary flow can show up in several different symptoms, such as difficulty starting the stream, reduced stream, incomplete emptying, dribbling, and frequent small squirts of a dammed-up bladder. This can amount to twenty or more trips to the men's room per day and a dozen or more times during the night."

"That sounds like no fun."

"Remember in the beginning how my symptoms were mild and crescendoed slowly? And for two years or more, I'd gotten up more often to go to the bathroom at night?"

"No kidding. But don't listen to me…oh, noooo…, just keep bulling ahead," she chided in mock admonition.

"Yeah, you were right for once."

"For once?" she grinned with exaggerated incredulity.

"OK, OK. So I convinced myself that those trips were simply the by-product of age. I know I'm bullheaded. Anyhow, as you know too well, I just blew off any doubts by saying 'I feel fine. It's just all the bike riding.'"

I went on to explain that when the inflammation arrived, it surely would show up during radiation treatments—the stinging, spasms, and burning could be substantial. I joked that I vowed to keep this in mind the next time I encountered an older guy in the men's room holding up the line at the urinal. If he were standing there with a sheepish grin and furrowed brow, he'd probably be thinking: "Damn it, prostate, don't fail me now." I would cut him a lot of slack because he'd be vexed enough as it was. In fact, he would be lucky not to soil his underwear in the action. A man in that position has long since stopped hoping for a stream. If he were suffering post-radiation prostatitis, from what I've heard, each urination event would be a mini-crisis. A few burning spasmodic squirts relieve only the moment's crisis. He forces them through by holding his breath and bearing down, like moving constipated stool. He's pushing to get the urine to flow past the inflamed prostatic urethra. It's called the Valsalva maneuver."

"Okay, so in English, the urine gets stopped up, so you have to push and pull and giggle to get something to come out. And you can poop your pants in the process."

"Ah, yes. That's about it."

Her eyes did glaze over as I got more into the teaching mode. The gist of it was as follows. To put such urinary symptoms in the context of the prostate, the clinical interpretation is not always simple. The problem could be acute prostatitis from infection or trauma (like prolonged biking), it might be benign prostatic enlargement (BPH), or it could be prostate cancer. Since the symptoms themselves are not completely specific and since those from cancer may not even surface for years, men over 50 should get an annual PSA blood test and have a digital rectal exam done by their doctor. These two simple tests, obtained at yearly or half-year intervals, will detect nearly three-quarters of all prostate cancers before they break free from the gland and spread to other parts of the body.

"Just like you did, right, Doc?"

119

"Yeah, I know. But let me finish."

I pressed on to elaborate on how once a cancer breaks free, it becomes a much more complicated picture. Once again, this cancer is like an iceberg—a man will never guess he has a problem, let alone realize its magnitude, until the tip surfaces. By that time there are urinary symptoms indicating significant mass effect.

"Stay with me, honey. Don't glaze over because you need to know this. It's two different ball games based on whether it has spread or stayed local. Obviously, we want local."

I continued by explaining that it even may have spread to bone or other body parts. In that case there would be pain or perhaps a stress fracture in a thinned bone. Sooner or later it would kill me. Therefore, the routine tests are crucial—they would tell us if I had a decent chance of survival, or a long shot, or none.

"There, was that so bad? You can come back, now, sweetheart. I just wanted to get it all straight out loud."

"It would have been better in English."

"I know. I just lapsed into my medical thing, probably to get some distance. After all, it may be killing me as I speak. Remember, the cells in the biopsy were described as aggressive bad boys. I don't know the workup yet."

"Yes, I know, sweetheart. You tell it in Chinese if you need to. All I want is for you to get a handle on it, however you can. And I'm sure you'll do it thoroughly. Just keep your chin up. So will I."

******

It was about that time, still within week one, that Polly's package arrived in the mail. It contained a note wishing me love and expressing her confidence that I would see it through. She also referred me to Man to Man, a self-help support group of men, for men, about prostate cancer—it's one of the only male support groups for a medical illness. There was a resource of information and support.

As I looked into the writings, I recognized once again that we men should take the lead from women about openly validating the human experience of contending with life-shattering traumas. We haven't said much, let alone written much, about our emotional journeys. I'd found many references written by women about breast cancer, for example. In fact, in the midst of many hundreds of female writers, I could find only a mere handful of men who have written about this male killer, and almost none dealt with the male emotional and spiritual aspects of the experience.

Man to Man, an outgrowth of the classic book by Michael Korda some ten years prior, has been one of the few examples of male attempts to do so. It's a national network of men supporting and educating other men about prostate cancer and offers written material, directs attention to resources, and provides small-group emotional support; wives and other loved ones also benefit. This is the real deal. I found its Web site by typing "Man to Man" into a search engine and by going to the Web site for the American Cancer Society for a Web connection and a toll-free number. I got some very helpful info at that site and met some supportive men in the local chapter. While sadly there has not been a men's movement analogous to that for women, I still took heart in that organization. It helped validate my becoming more open to direct caring from men—no small feat for "Superdoc."

******

121

That conversation with Susan was about as far as I wanted to push the information barrage. I had told her the generalities. Now, sitting at what had become my familiar spot at my desk, reading the computer screen, and making notes, I compiled for myself a summary of the specifics.

In short, if the cancer was localized, surgery would get it over with, but the downtime could be considerable and some side effects could occasionally be permanent. Also, if it was localized, I could go for radiation oncology; the downtime would be nil but there would be four to six months of active treatment and plenty of fallout after that. Of course, if it had metastasized, all bets were off and I would need an estate attorney. But no matter what the side effects, the one I surely didn't want was death.

I had learned that, for men, this is their silent killer. Of all the cancers, prostate is the second most common, behind lung cancer. It strikes 1 in 5 men over age sixty and kills 27,000 of us every year, and it affects many more who survive. This has only come to light in the last few decades, perhaps reflecting a real increase due to some environmental factors but also likely as a function of increased longevity and increased accuracy of testing. I'm told that this cancer can take hold in a man after he reaches the age of 50 and often moves slowly. It's virtually certain that when life spans were shorter and detection methods less accurate, many men died from other causes. Anyhow, that info was only of academic interest. I needed practical material for my case.

As I started my research, I had tools unavailable just a decade before—the Internet and the World Wide Web. In 1993 or before, who would've reacted to news of prostate cancer by saying "Let's see what we can find on the Web?" At least not old-timers like me who grew up without computers.

This vast new resource has both good information and bad; therefore, I'd come to learn that it's best to approach with caution. Some people put up bad information out of ignorance, and occasionally someone posts blatantly false advice out of malice and mischief. Nevertheless, there are many useful sites that tell you about medical options and about complementary treatments.

The Web has become a tool of choice in so many everyday decisions that it has seemed automatic for many to search it for help in crises. Often, it has been helpful for me, but I've always had a healthy skepticism until I know the source. Had it come from people, organizations, or institutions I recognized? Otherwise, I've taken the information with a grain of salt (and sometimes pounds of salt). Quotes that appear to be endorsements can be quoted from anywhere on any site, so the speaker may or may not have endorsed the site.

One rule of thumb I've used has been to stick with known commodities—in medicine that would mean the health care providers whose reputations are established. Many hospitals have developed excellent Web sites, as have most medical schools. The National Institutes of Health (NIH) has been another good place for me to look; the same has been the case for many organizations whose reputations long predate the Internet: the American Cancer Society, the American Heart Association, and the one already mentioned, Man to Man. They've been good for years, with sound quality control and with links to other reliable sites. Still, I've borne in mind the admonition "Reader beware."

With those caveats in mind, I approached my PC. My trusty browser identified many thousands of entries on the prostate, and I went through them until the information became repetitive. In short, here is a brief summary of what I learned, which I read and reread several times for days.

An evaluation, or workup, always involves some combination of laboratory tests on various bodily fluids, as well as X-rays, scans, and magnetic resonance imaging (MRI). In the case of prostate cancer, the workup should include a PSA, a chemistry profile, a complete blood count, a digital rectal exam (DRE), and an ultrasound with biopsy.

When I reached the point of some of the more elaborate or technical diagnostic or treatment techniques, geography started to determine options. In some areas, hospitals don't always have state-of-the-art equipment. This is a particular concern in the field of detection, where the newer the equipment, like color flow Doppler, the better picture you get of a cancer.

Luckily, Sarasota had several experienced urologists and radiology oncologists whose technology is state-of-the-art, some of which includes 3D color flow Doppler, which shows the blood supply to the cancer and surrounding tissues. My own Doppler study showed an early attempt by the cancer to breech the capsule around the gland (not good). A total body bone scan looks for metastases (the spreading of the cancer into bones and other organs), and a pelvic scan gives a more focused picture of areas near the source. For me, both studies were normal, so I took a deep breath. The Reaper scowled, lowered his scythe, and moved toward the background. At least my odds were in the ballpark.

Some hospitals or clinics provide MRI examination of not just the pelvis but also the prostate itself by using a rectal core magnet, which feels very intrusive and as big as a watermelon. Trust me--that one was no fun, but thankfully, for all the trouble, mine was negative. The Reaper frowned and moved farther back. But the experience reminded me of the intrusion and discomfort that patients go through as part of their workup and receive little attention thereafter, even when they complain.

The rest of the testing was painless. That was even true of the biopsy, which made the diagnosis and preceded the fancy workup. Though it involved shooting a hollow needle through the rectal wall into several areas in the gland, the discomfort was so minimal that afterward I went straight back to the office. Some doctors do more sophisticated blood tests. Mine did some having to do with the endocrine blood parameters and prostrate proteins.

Sometimes during this kind of intellectual research, I would pause to wipe away a tear of irony at being so thoroughly medical about a process that was working inside of me, trying to kill me as I sat there. For all my talk of growing up and getting proactive, I still at times had nagging doubts about my impotence in the face of the mystery.

Is all this time at the computer worth the effort? Is it just busywork to fill the time between now and when I languish in a nursing home? Here I am, proceeding full steam ahead as if there really are moves to make that can reverse the tide and save me.

Without a single guarantee, am I just kidding myself?

******

With no viable alternative, I shoved back down the doubts and terror and proceeded to put together a condensed listing of the options I weighed:

- Watch and wait. If one is very old, one may outlive it. If it's widely metastasized, the choices narrow considerably. The treatments for these advanced

125

complications can be more arduous and even more harmful than the disease itself. The physician will weigh all the factors with the patient.

- External beam radiation therapy (EBRT). A few places in the country offer highly sophisticated stereotaxic EBRT, some instances of which can be very sophisticated four-dimensional image guided radiation therapy (4D IG-IMRT). The radiation can be delivered to precise points in space without going through—and damaging—surrounding tissue. The computer even adjusts for breathing movements. The treatments take ten minutes and are delivered five days per week, for five weeks. This treatment itself will likely deplete your energy somewhat and produce annoying urinary symptoms, but these are no big deal.

- Surgery. If cancer is localized, total prostatectomy gets it over and done with but on rare occasion risks dispersing the cancer cells and even leaving behind some cancer cells, not to mention the unlikely possibility of permanent impotence and/or incontinence. There is also a partial excision available through a periscope-like tube (laparoscope), with removal of tissue with less blood loss than with surgery.

- Cryotherapy. The method of cryotherapy kills cancer cells in a localized spot by freezing them to death.

- Androgen blockade. Androgens are male hormones, and this is a fancy way of describing testosterone shutdown, or chemical castration. Since the male hormone (testosterone) feeds prostate cancer cells, its absence starves them. Medications such as Casodex and Proscar are blocking agents, which thwart the ability of testosterone and its derivatives from reaching cancer receptors; Lupron turns off testosterone production. Together, these drugs turn the estrogen/testosterone balance upside down. As a result, a man becomes feminized with abnormal levels of estrogen. This is often called "the andropause."

Welcome to "eunuch-hood."

On come the hot flashes, sweats, painfully enlarged breasts, fatigue, and early to bed. And a man won't soon forget the loss of sexual feeling or function. Thankfully, this pretty much reverses after treatment stops, but the recovery can take a year or more. The side-effect picture varies with the individual—and with the duration of treatment—from a few months of modest symptoms to a year or more (even two) of brisk symptoms. My aftermath was at the extreme end of the spectrum, I've been told. One's wife may have little sympathy for some aspects, pointing out that every woman goes through such menopausal symptoms. But castration status, however temporary, likely won't be any more fun for her than it will be for the man with the nonfunctioning gonads.

☐Seed implants. The implants typically require an overnight stay in the hospital. The number of seeds may vary, going up to a hundred or more. Many medical centers and hospitals place them while the patient is under regional anesthesia, which takes a Star Wars–like precision technology. Then as the post-radiation prostatitis roars on, the ball game has really begun. Painful, frequent, and sparse urination feels like squirts of burning hot tacks thirty or more times a day.

I wanted to avoid surgery for several reasons. It was important to me to keep working; aside from the fact that my patients didn't need an interruption in treatment, I didn't want to give up my day-to-day work. I love my work and I knew it would help me keep up my morale. I believed that I could pull off keeping my own agenda way in the background, at least during practice hours. Surgery would have entailed several weeks or more of recovery—time when sessions with patients would not have been possible.

There were also the risk factors. In surgery, there would have been a small chance that I might become permanently incontinent or left with erectile dysfunction. The course I chose entailed some predictable problems, but primarily temporary ones.

Radiation oncology was the alternative I chose. Specifically, I decided to combine three options: overlapping androgen blockade, external beam radiation (EBRT), and seed implants. The androgen blockade was to begin simultaneously with external radiation and run four months; this five-week course of stereotaxic radiation was to be followed by the seed implantation procedure. Overall, it was to be a four- to five-month aggressive course against an aggressive cancer.

I realized that choices between treatments for life-threatening illnesses seldom are between something nice and something uncomfortable. I was facing a decision between options that were painful and those that were more painful. But, hey, I was dealing with life or death, so degrees of discomfort and functional side effects were small considerations. It was my sense that radiation oncology had the edge, even for localized disease—a decision I would never get to test because there was only one shot.

******

Nearly a week had passed since cancer day, and my

head was filled with information. I hung my legs over the end of the dock, letting my feet barely touch the water as I meditated on the options and a decision. Even though my workup was unfinished, the options boiled down to small differences in outcome data, likely side effects, and downtime. I didn't know at the time that even with successful treatment for nonmetastatic disease, the aftermath of my side effects would stretch out two years, though I wouldn't be down and out.

I gazed out over the still lagoon shimmering in the bright moonlight. Occasional crashes from under the mangroves overhanging the perimeter signaled feeding snook. I grinned at the thought of fishing for those wily and powerful shallow-water game fish in area bays and inlets.

Have I done the last of that?

With a deep breath, I set my reflection on the week's events.

I've seen life's routine pitches, fastballs, curves, and sinkers, and I've taken some dings. I've hit a few and missed a few. What I hadn't realized was that I'd been set up perfectly for the beanball. Life stood out on the mound, kicked, and threw, and the pitch was pure heat, straight for me: the phone call with the biopsy results, when my carefully constructed world cracked. I might've paid attention when the last couple of pitches whizzed by my head, but I'd barely noticed them. There'd been a couple of years of extra trips to the bathroom at night. But hey...that one went right by me. Even the high PSA level hadn't dented my attitude.

I'd kept my optimism and stayed in the batter's box, so to speak. Others might've called it denial, but for me, it was just my long-held positive attitude of staying with the challenge. After all, I knew this pitcher, didn't I? Wasn't he the one who gave out all the free passes or the straight fastballs down the middle?

That's a corny way to describe being caught so off guard that it prodded surprising outrage and disillusionment from my core. I was scared as hell, so I got into gear. I decided to go for the X-rays and temporary eunuch-hood, hoping that there had been no spread. If there had been, I'd have made the same choice anyway.

******

My treatment plan was set. Now I had to follow through and stay the course, come what may. That would require more than the medical treatments; it would demand that I do my part. I needed to bring my readiness and resilience—physically, emotionally, and spiritually. All of that would require conscious and proactive cultivation. Therefore, I had to design a plan of my own contribution to get on top of my game and stay there. I had most of the necessary knowledge about prostate cancer in my head and was learning more. Beyond that, it would be up to me. Implementation on a daily basis was going to be imperative.

Chapter 11
Physical Requirements

Life boiled down to fifteen-minute intervals, diapers, urinals, public restrooms, pocketed pride. I stayed fit with diet, exercise, and meditation. Side effects were draining enough, and I didn't need aggravation from bad habits.

It turned out that I had localized cancer. The treatment I'd chosen, a combination of temporary castration with androgen blockade, external radiation, and internal seed implants, came with a list of side effects. Pooling all sources, it looked like I would be contending with many discomforts, let alone inconveniences. Little did I realize at the outset just how daunting the side effects would prove to be. What choice did I have? Die then and there?

Unfazed, I took as cool a look as possible at the specifics and decided that I'd better make allowances in my schedule for frequent pees, especially at odd times. And I promised myself that, if at all possible, I would maintain my daily workouts and full clinical schedule. If I had to adjust...well, then I would at the time. But my initial posture was to keep up the basics of my life structure. Little did I know at the outset how challenging that would be. In fact, thank God for my unflappable optimism. I walked into a shit storm, whistling.

Acid diets feed cancer, at least according to my research. That was the diet I and most Americans loved, with lots of carbs, sweets, meats, fried foods, and dairy products. Alkaline diets, on the other hand, were said to be anticancer, but those are the ones only a handful of dedicated health nuts can abide. The alkaline diets emphasized green vegetables and non-sugary fruits—I called it the "Bugs Bunny Diet." But again, the alternative wasn't savory, so out went the meats, pasta, pizza, and lots of my usual fare. And no wine or beer. I drank powdered grasses and veggies every morning and began using only distilled water. Lo and behold, I even started to lose weight.

******

Skulking down the personal hygiene aisle at the pharmacy, I spotted the adult diapers and the insert absorbent pads for my underwear. Just like when I was fifteen and sneaking a peak at the new *Playboy* on the shelf, I darted over to the items, and as I furtively looked about for horrified expressions, I deftly snatched a few boxes of each and cradled them in my arms. I hoped that enough jacket material largely hid them from glances that would've screamed, "There goes another geezer with his diapers." By the time I reached the checkout, it was like I was still sixteen, buying a condom from the seventeen-year-old female cashier. I would've liked to have crouched down out of sight behind the counter and just reached up high enough to hand over the money.

Just as I exited the store, I exploded with laughter and could hardly wait to tell Susan. She added insult to injury by saying that I could have saved some money by just buying plain old sanitary napkins and stuffing them into my jockey shorts. We both roared at the absurdity of it all.

I stocked up, quickly storing a stash in both of our cars, our home, and all three offices. And as if I hadn't endured enough chagrin in the store, I remembered the plastic urinals when I got to the parking lot. So back in I went, revisiting in my mind the condom and skin magazine purchases all over again, this time exiting with three urinals. I could only guess what the young clerk's fantasy was upon seeing the same old fart reappear, carrying not one but three plastic receptacles. Anyhow, one urinal went in each car and one went to the bedside.

Speaking of sleep arrangements, I knew from the start that Susan's light sleeping habits would never tolerate being awakened many times at night as I rose to pee—my snoring had been adjustment enough—so I relocated to the guest bedroom. It had its own bathroom attached, so the trip from the bed would be short. Most importantly, she would not be disturbed. One of the mortifying urinals sat on the bedside table, reminding me not just of prostate cancer but also more generally of age's inevitable toll on functions that are taken for granted until they're messed up. The diapers didn't help any. For more than a few moments, I felt older than I was.

I knew that frequent urinations would require redesign of the time structure of all aspects of my life. Appointments could likely last no more than thirty minutes, so my schedule was reset accordingly, except for some tasks that required more time; for those, I would excuse myself halfway through. Driving to and from work would probably be okay as long as the trips fell within the thirty-minute window, and the same would go for any driving for social or entertainment purposes. It was to be quick trips, no trips, or trips interrupted by strategic men's rooms. I scoped out the gas stations along common routes in Sarasota and carried my safety valve urinal just in case.

When I taught one-hour (or longer) conferences, participated in depositions, or attended unavoidably long meetings, I would ask for or simply suggest a stretch break for "fanny fatigue" or "calls to nature." As it turned out, that seemed to work, but I occasionally got the private giggles at the thought of how personal biology trumps even the most earnest of discussions.

Workouts at the gym fit easily with the twenty-to-thirty minute time intervals; besides, I could take breaks when ever I needed to. So they were to continue uninterrupted six days per week as always. My energy seemed about normal, especially at that early time of the day. But I wondered how I would hold up when the treatment side effects began to hit their height in the third and fourth months (January and February). Frankly, the information I had gleaned was general and contained the usual "blah, blah" about individual variation and so forth. So this would be an adventure with only a sketchy map.

My staff was with the program of my living in time bites, and each one of them was wonderful in making sure my appointments would be set to last no longer than thirty minutes. Not once was there ever a wisecrack about what was coming—the walk down the hall to the men's room. They knew when to be humorous and when not to be.

As I had expected from my research ahead of time, some aspects of personal life would have to change. Susan and I decided to forgo that winter season's tickets to the theater and symphony. For the few tickets that she already held in hand, she decided to go with a friend. We both agreed that my shuffling down the row of seats in front of patrons contorting themselves to get out of my way while I stepped on their toes was not going to happen. No apologies would have offset the rudeness.

And besides, I'd be just too embarrassed. In a two- or three-hour production, I'd have had to run the gauntlet four or five times. No way.

So we would confine our socializing to early evenings with friends at our home or theirs. Little did I realize at that planning stage just how much twenty-five dreaded trips to the bathroom were going to take from my energy by the end of each day—not to mention another twenty trips straight through the evening and night. We just considered the list of expected side effects and started making adjustments, expecting an average dose of trouble.

As for diet, I'd already started the rabbit diet. I decided to modify that a bit to include some grains and nuts, along with tofu, chicken, and seafood, but stayed away from alcohol, sweets, and fried foods. I just hoped that the flip-flop of my endocrine system wouldn't cause me to put on weight. Continued exercise and attention to diet should suffice, I thought. Little did I know.

Susan and I understood that my libido and manly function were to be interrupted. For how long, who knew? Sleeping apart had already been agreed on for the sake of my nightly treadmill every half hour to the bathroom, so there was just another interruption in our way of being with each other. We would just have to content ourselves with cuddling, kissing, and hugging, but as we had joked a hundred times already, "It beats the box."

In the past twenty years or so, I'd been an early riser and attentive to getting enough sleep, so there would be no need to rethink times of retiring and arising. In fact, my early-to-bed, early-to-rise routine had been the butt of jokes for years. At every New Year's Eve party, one of my friends—Paul—would inevitably nail me by asking for a toast at 10:00 P.M. "so Bob can go home to bed."

Faced with the prospect of many pees throughout the night, however, I anticipated trouble. Just how much trouble, however, I could not have predicted at that point, but I was willing to take a nightly sleeping pill if necessary, at least Sunday through Thursday night. Thankfully, there was one I was willing to use since it was commonly used for months at a stretch without apparent habituation or hangover. I would decide at the time.

******

So much for anticipating the practical and physical aspects. Staying on top also meant knowing appropriate ways to cope emotionally and spiritually as well as the hazards to avoid. Again, that was going to require conscious thought. No approach would just happen and then stay in place. I would need to walk myself all the way through the rocky journey, always trying to avoid making matters worse for myself. In effect, I was to be my own guide. To do that effectively and lovingly, I knew that I must meditate and reflect every day. In fact, I knew full well that unless coping responses to crisis get conscious attention, they can reflect the worst in us, not the best. That was not going to happen, so more thought and implementation.

Chapter 12

Emotional Tasks

The Serenity Prayer, the Rule of Holes, love and humor. My choice: Survive or live.

Another office day ended toward the end of the second week. The workup had told me that I was likely dealing with localized cancer. True, it was just starting to breech the capsule, but I may have caught it in time. To say the least, there was some relief in that much. My mind-set could therefore focus on dealing with treatments and side effects rather than with an inexorable, slowly spreading cancer takeover.

I paused for a few moments in my office wingback chair to reflect on the various patients who had asked me to help with all manner of human ills and troubles. I knew I could always learn something or at least be inspired. That day, three patients had presented with undiagnosed bipolar II disorder, several with depression, and many with adjustment reactions; most required attention to medication and some counseling. In general, the experience had been satisfying in that most were on the mend or soon would be. I was struck at how much more than ever I was aware of the frailty of life and the courage required for those valiant souls to make the best of it when they felt like they were falling apart. And in the midst of their distress, they had dared to ask me—at first a stranger—to help. My patients had often shown amazing human resilience. But even into the second week after my cancer diagnosis, at a personal level I was even more keenly aware than ever of the Great Mystery and the universality of its maddening demands.

But I was not seduced into distraction by some lofty reflection of the human condition—my life was on the line. My priority was to save it or to do the best I could by it. So I shifted from marveling at my patients' courage to the lessons they had taught me, the practical dos and don'ts about coping effectively. I'd witnessed enough triumphs and botches to know what to strive for and what to avoid.

Two weeks prior, flummoxed on the beach, I'd determined to get to the truth in order to be grounded and in charge of myself. That was rule number one, and the conviction continued. But there were other principles taught by thousands of my patients: an acceptance mirrored in the Serenity Prayer, the power of love and humor, and the role of personal myth in replaying history (especially the script we thought had been left behind but which had hung on just out of awareness). There were many more concepts that comprised mature, effective coping. It was my time to put these into action for my own survival.

******

So I asked myself what was unique in my cancer

response and what was generalized. Even more interesting for me, probably because of my profession, was the question of what path I had taken to get there. I started to wonder, somewhat rhetorically.

Why was I, who should have known better, so thrown for a loop? Was that what anybody would go through—at least initially—when their life was in jeopardy? And even if it were, how was it that I happened to be in that position of naiveté? And did it warrant all the introspection I recently had been devoting to it?

Again, I had to reassure myself that it did, that this wasn't just an exercise to quell my apparent fragility. So I began to look at the origin of most of my reactions—my development, my story. I wanted to be clear about what in my story had set me up to rise so high and fall off a cliff.

That metaphor's just a bit dramatic, Bobby Boy. OK, then why did I feel the child-like outrage? Was it an offense to my unbridled confidence and optimism? I never thought I was that self-absorbed or foolish, but maybe I had been...deep down. Anyhow, being positive is a good thing. No hope, no life. I'm living proof that hoping and taking chances too often bring unplanned hurt at the most unjust times. There was the Great Mystery again.

I was undoubtedly like many patients whose myths had evolved from—and been reinforced by—life experiences from childhood on. Some were happy and some very sad, but most were mixtures. After all, even for those who lived fully, there was always some sense of being unexpectedly shocked, of being caught off guard, by a personal loss or health disaster, and there were usually some elements of their having had a hand in their own tragedy.

Hell, that's been much of my work.

In my case, parental adoration and expectations engendered confidence and optimism in me. But as I had

139

recently discovered, it appeared to come with a price tag—
a naïve sense of being charmed and entitled to a pass. As
hard as it is to admit, I felt bulletproof—the kind of
invincibility all adolescents believe in. Apparently I hadn't
fully outgrown mine, but I was determined to do so since I
knew I wasn't compelled to endlessly relive my history. I
could change the script, and cancer woke me up in a hurry
and gave me that chance.

I decided that I would spend some time in my Sarasota
office pulling together a kind of psychological plan of how
to approach this disaster. I would use all that I had learned
from experience and would go beyond platitudes of
"personal best" and "positive attitude." For one thing, I
wanted to get a hold on what had kept me in denial and
innocence for so long. I'd already delved into that in the
first few days when I meditated on Mom and Dad, who
were my roots for better and worse. So I went back for
more.

Of course I'd paid the price of my star myth through the
years, but extra pounds and the like were not the most
expensive costs. Possibly the dearest of all was the failure
to get a routine PSA. So that part of my story screamed out
for insight and correction.

I slouched back, took deep breaths as I loosened my tie,
and zoned out into thought. A panorama came to mind,
composed of the many personal odysseys of my patients. I
applied the same approach to myself. I knew well that most
began with some mythology that took hold from childhood
and continued into maturity. Often my patients would be
saddled with some kind of defining family role they had
bought into, such as that of "loser," or "jerk," or "clown,"
or "Mother Earth," just like I had been. Some went on to
happy outcomes; others did not. Mine wasn't looking so
bad compared to some, but it was still encumbering when

the cancer crisis hit.

As I had learned from my work, it was always important to keep in mind that a myth need not be permanent. It may look like an integral part of someone's life cycle, but it was not indelible.

In fact, if that weren't so, I wouldn't have a profession.

I've seen many patients find the ingredients to overcome the past. Some call it being reborn or saved; others call it personal growth. My patients who were introspective were always curious about ways to improve themselves emotionally, intellectually, and spiritually. That's why they and I could do what we did day in and day out.

As for my story, it seemed rather ordinary compared to many others, but it compelled scrutiny and change if I was to get through this death threat effectively. This kind of reflection wasn't self-indulgence, any more than were the memories prompted by calls to Dave and DK. All of my history had made me what I was to that day. Some of it had been triumphantly successful, at least in my little world, and some had been humorously naïve and immature. Some formative elements came from my adolescent disappointments and embarrassments that lingered into adulthood; some factors had been a little boy's fantasy of being such a good little star that he'd get a pass, that his prayer would be granted for his dearest wish, that he'd get through life unscathed just like he had in his youth. The beach walk on diagnosis day brought out that nonsense in spades, and that impairment must not continue. Indeed, such dysfunctional elements might turn out to be the instrument of my death, for all I knew.

After all, only God's prompting, not mine, got me to the lab for a PSA.

141

******

Sitting there in my office, I let my thoughts wander to a woman whom I had seen that day. She had been an inspiration I could learn from, though over time her straits had been more dire than mine. Although she wasn't facing a bullet coming toward her in slow motion, she had taught me a lot about bouncing back from what, in her case, seemed overwhelming odds. Her story should remind me of the way that some elements of personality take over, in spite of what we know we should do, and run our life for worse, not better. It's the source of the well-worn expression about being one's own worst enemy. But I knew from thousands of examples that one could turn that around and be a part of saving oneself.

Mrs. Morris had often considered leaving, but Mr. Morris had told her he would kill her if she did. It was only when their 15-year-old daughter revealed her father's sexual abuse that Mrs. M. finally contacted the local women's shelter. That had been the last straw. They advised her and she made her plan. One night, after Mr. Morris had passed out in a drunken stupor, mother and daughter snuck out of the house, gathered up the baggage they'd hidden under the front stoop, and drove to the secret shelter. Their ultimate goal was Florida, with the promise of a new life.

A few months later Mrs. Morris came to my office with a referral from the Sarasota Women's Shelter. She was worn down physically from her years of abuse as well as her recent upheaval. She'd had the courage to move to a strange new place, but she had no job, friends, or relatives; she just had her daughter. Her sadness and stress had been diagnosed as "depression," but she had refused antidepressants, wanting to rely only on her grit and her faith. Despite all of this, Mrs. M. was neither cynical nor demoralized. She had a heart of gold and a firm faith that no terror could squash. She needed support and didn't want medication if it could be avoided.

Mrs. M. had endured all of this alone for several reasons: Her parents had died when she was sixteen; she had relatives, but they gave up on her when she wouldn't leave her abusive husband, because they had no understanding of the dynamics of domestic violence and imprisonment; her husband had isolated her, keeping her from any people or agencies that might have helped. She'd taken refuge in long hours on the job, but that left her home chaotic and unfit for visitors. The one thing she had maintained was her faith in God, so she prayed daily, went to church on Sunday, and read her Bible at night, after her husband passed out.

Just six months after relocating here, Mrs. M.'s daughter committed suicide. She had fallen victim to posttraumatic stress and depression, and rather than accepting treatment, she had thrown herself into a fast crowd of older teens whose lives revolved around drugs and the mall—so-called mall rats. One late night, drunk and tripping, she had climbed into a warm bath and slit her wrists. Mrs. M. found her in the morning.

We slowly worked our way through her grief and her feelings of guilt at having "failed" all three of her children. That unrealistic sense of responsibility took some undoing. For an entrapped victim, she had in fact gone 99 percent of the way for all three—albeit at too much of a cost to herself and at the expense of maintenance of the dangerous status quo. Through all of it, she held tight to her faith. She had the remarkable ability to allow for a larger plan, however obscure it seemed. In a time when she had no friends to talk to, her faith sustained her, and not once did she talk of taking her own life. She cried and castigated herself but never fell into frank clinical depression. It may have been her own miracle, but she never required the medication she so wanted to avoid. She prayed many times every day. She found a local church, threw herself into a job, and did volunteer work for the Women's Center.

Mrs. M. saved herself through the power of faith and her own grit. Often I had difficulty holding back my tears as she told me about her long years of trauma. Her tenacity alone was impressive enough, but her ability to hold onto her goodwill and generosity boggled my mind. It was people like Mrs. M. who taught me about courage, faith, and love. She unknowingly added to my own growth as a man. These days I draw on it with admiration and gratitude. If only I could muster that kind of resilience...

While her life story was an extreme one, I thought about it to illustrate one end of the spectrum of trauma. Her heartache was readily understandable, and her survival was heroic. My other patients have provided me with many more stories, often being more ordinary in their severity but having in common the human experience of trying to find meaning and purpose in the face of the Great Mystery, especially when reeling from a hit.

Their unsung courage and persistence have always amazed me. The stories were usually less extreme than that of Mrs. M. No matter. Every man and woman had to show up every day and contend with what was on their plate, do their best, and put on a face for the world. Mrs. M. was hardly the only one, but her story came to mind at that moment probably because it was so dire. Maybe I was in that kind of mind-set because the Grim Reaper loomed.

******

I sat reflecting on the complexities of personal history and our power to change it—to save ourselves. In that moment I thought of Willie Sutton's focus on getting to the heart of the matter and going where truth and love are. In fact, I often thought about that.

Over years of practice I'd had the privilege of witnessing people with faith courageously overcoming traumas: One sixty-five-year-old man had suffered two heart attacks and lung cancer; another man was knocked senseless by the deaths of his wife and children in a car wreck; one woman I'd treated successfully for lifelong attention deficit disorder returned after a nine-month hiatus, clarifying her absence by telling of her recent out-of-the-blue diagnosis of inoperable brain cancer; still another man reeled from job loss, bankruptcy, and prostate cancer. The heroic stories went on and on. Especially since my own bomb dropped, I often wondered: How would I have held up if I'd had to face challenges like those? Those people and many like them had managed to get through each day on a steady diet of love and faith, keeping them just positive enough to carry on. On both personal and professional levels, their recognition of faith's power was clear.

The variety of these tales illustrated that I shared with them the tasks of living, regardless of specific gifts and curses. It was clearer than ever that, as a friend had told me, making the most of the hand we've been dealt is the name of the game. I knew that such resilience wasn't limited to faith and love, but it surely required them both. There were additional coping skills to review, so I pressed on.

In those first tender weeks post-diagnosis, I could hardly help but acknowledge that while the landscape of life itself might have been largely uncontrollable, the path through it was not. My job was to find mine right now. I was bound to make this journey at the very least a learning experience. And I didn't mean a head trip; I meant maturation for whatever time I had left. So there was a place for dos and don'ts, pushed and maintained by love and faith...and don't forget humor.

******

I had come to believe that the human body and spirit have a natural healing inclination that, when nurtured by loving compassion and directed by the right insights and skills, would go about its business of mending, so I needed to clear the way and keep it passable. That, in a nutshell, was part of what I was trying to do in all my introspection.

As for the faith component, I often had meditated and reflected about how central faith in God is, however it is experienced. I surely did during this crisis time, reminding myself that faith may take form in any of the world's orthodox religions or may manifest itself in private mysticism or love of nature, such as I'd recently been experiencing. It didn't matter what one called it; it was simply an understanding that life has a connection to the Big Energy, the Divine. Mine was pretty much private.

Mrs. M. believed in Jesus, attended church, and read the Bible. I've known this to be true of many people of faith, but I've also known many whose spiritual lives were private. They, like I, expressed their faith in meditation. They might have found the most comfort in practicing their devotion at the beach or in their homes. My sacred places have been home, office, and hospital. Nature and music have always been good for my soul, but the actual places have been those three. Formal orthodoxy hasn't been a requirement because regardless of form or packaging, the essence of faith is spirituality itself. While the external structure was helpful for some, it was unnecessary for others, me included.

So, I thought, the long and short of it is that love and faith would heal and maintain my heart and soul and would do the same for my body to the extent that was possible. Was this desperate foxhole fervor? I hoped not. Instead, I saw my awakening as a constructive response to a jolt.

After countless hours in my tree house room and my other lovely offices, I came to realize that knowing one's heart doesn't always come naturally. Indeed, that's an understatement. For years, I've gone through each day attending to dozens of surface concerns, the details of job, children, housekeeping, and recreation. They've dominated most of my waking moments just as they have everyone else's. Quiet reflection could easily have been the forgotten stepchild, if it had not been made part of my daily care routine. Hardball introspection takes hard work, so it doesn't just happen, even for knowledgeable and psychologically minded people...even for therapists. I gratefully recognized that I, for one, had always known the importance of the daily ritual of introspection. But now, more than in usual times, it was imperative.

In my case, I had knowledge, training, and confidence along with a positive attitude and faith. But I also had my myth's naïve omnipotence and its hazardous blindness. That was the naiveté that had set me up for being blindsided. As I thought about the big picture, however, maybe the entire journey had been necessary for this life— the rises, the falls, and the rebirths.

Oh, spare me. Can you sound any more cliché, Professor Superdoc? Try "plain-speak." Yes, it probably is the way lives continually evolve to higher and more enlightened levels—a step at a time. Anyway, that's the way mine seems to have shifted.

147

The general principle again struck me: Unacknowledged stuff keeps one stuck. It didn't keep me entirely stalled, but it sure set me up with a soft side I wasn't fully aware of. So that's where the bullet struck.

That's why, like Willie said, total truth was required.

******

Before closing up and heading for home, I allowed recollection of one other patient I had seen that day, Tom N. His story embodied a problematic way of handling his unpleasant feelings. In fact, his picture was so dysfunctional that it was instructive as to how not to operate. Until he changed, he had been out of touch with his soft, or vulnerable, side. He truly was acting like the agent of his own demise. I respectfully held out his story as a reminder of the Rule of Holes, or how to shoot oneself in the foot.

Tom was fifty-one by the time I was asked to consult on his case in the hospital. His wife was fed up with his anger and gave him an ultimatum to seek help, so he acquiesced to his doctor's suggestion. He was a hulking red-faced man who, at the very sight of me, started on a tirade about nurses, hospital food, back pain, and his own foolishness in having climbed up on one roof too many. He lay immobilized in an orthopedic contraption. Yet with all his vitriol, I sensed terrible heartache rather than rage.

I reviewed his biologically based disorders. I considered bipolar disorder or other possible causes for such a disturbed temperament. His history showed that, as a rule, Tom hadn't been moody or irritable, and his motor didn't run fast and slow; he had no known genetic predisposition for mood disorders. He described himself as usually a pleasant, hardworking guy and thought of himself as well liked unless he was crossed or was faced with a crisis. Then all hell broke loose.

He recalled how he had lashed out at those close to him upon the death of his father five years earlier. He'd also done it when his wife was diagnosed with breast cancer three years later and again when his daughter lost an eye in a freak skiing accident and when his son got himself arrested and jailed for dealing weed. It sounded as if Tom saw the best defense as being a good offense. He couldn't bring himself to grieve, so he bellowed.

He knew that his guilt over the excesses had curbed some of his overt anger, and he also realized that there was some kind of block to normal grief. He understood this much because, during these crises, he could feel in his heart of hearts a terrible and bottomless sorrow trying to well up. It terrified him, so he squashed it with outrage at those around him. His wife had tried to talk with him each time he sidetracked into rage, but he knew the drill. He was bright and surprisingly psychologically minded—it was as if he knew better but just couldn't make good on it.

The final blow came when Tom fell off his roof while trying to repair a satellite dish, an accident which laid him low here in the hospital bed, back broken, career threatened, while he struggled to contain his anger at this last bomb. He wondered if he could be cursed. Was this the punishment for his "anger problem"? He couldn't help but be nasty to the nurses. Life had become a cascade of unfair losses and burdens. His eyes swelled with unreleased tears. I sensed a profound sadness and heartbreak, but all I saw on the surface was rage—the words didn't match the music.

I listened to his outbursts and then heard him out as he attempted to explain his take on the situation. We established a connection, and that's when I felt it was time to shift to the heart of the matter. Tom was all too ready.

With empathic support, I went straight for his grieving heart—it was the right move at the right moment. He opened up the flood gates, and out poured all of his sorrows, betrayals, and abandonments, both current and old. It wasn't as if he suddenly could handle these emotions; rather, it was the opening of an emotional abscess. The pus flowed, so to speak, starting the healing process. My own heart ached for him as I accompanied him through the beginnings of his transition from a raging bull to a weeping, bereft man.

In further consultations, both in the hospital, and later in my office, Tom explored his life story to discover when and how he had begun avoiding heartache. There had been no room for sadness in his family: His mother was stoic, while his father raged. He followed his father's example of suppressing the "soft" side of himself and contrived a myth: "Better mad than sad." Framed on his desk was a sign that said: "Just when you thought things couldn't get worse, they did." This pessimistic wisecrack didn't leave much room for hope.

Over time, Tom learned to see his dysfunctional echoes and his pattern of avoiding normal sadness. He came to acknowledge disappointment and grief as part of life's palette, and these became a part of his normal response to crises. He saw that he'd been paying a price greater than that of the problem. These insights became usable only when he opened up his heart. With that healing under way, he gained confidence in his capacity to bear sorrow; with all of his important emotional responses on the table, he could roll with the punches and use what he knew. He didn't have to hide from his scary feelings, he stopped shaking his fist at the heavens, and he gave up his cynicism. His way became easier to live with. His wife was pleased and grateful.

I recalled Tom's story, along with others like it, as I looked into myself and talked with my heart. If I was going to deal with cancer competently, I had to face my fears. A Star is never comfortable with helplessness. A doctor at the top of his form won't have an easy time with impotence of any kind; after all, he's the caregiver, right? Yet I had to live with these things and accept them for what they were. I had to learn the skills that my patients had developed. I was blessed to have them as models.

There was a bit of Tom N. in my star nonsense. Though I didn't rage like he did, we shared the myth of self-sufficiency during a crisis. Our self-reliance worked fine free of crisis, but when it hit the fan, we bionic men reverted to hiding behind old defenses. Tom shot himself in the foot in obvious ways; I was more subtle. He yelled; I rationalized and asked for less. He beat on scapegoats (including himself), while I politely turned into myself, cooking up some pasta and seasoning the sauce with psychobabble.

I'm sure it was always transparent to Susan. When I hurt, she never failed to help me pull out the sadness hidden beneath my star façade. But I hadn't needed much pulling or tugging to see this cancer threat. My reactions were bursting out all over and I kept them coming. I just needed her loving support.

But thank God for small blessings. At least I didn't have to deal with the old male myth that big boys don't cry. Despite my Superdoc mentality, I'd never been too scared to show vulnerability. I was open and ready for whatever emotions were to come.

******

That was enough for one day, but the reminders had

been worth staying for. I welcomed any clarity in those early days of preparing myself to take on treatment. I promised myself to stay in close touch with how I really felt, to stay connected to my loved ones, and to continue to find the irony and humor in this crazy, wonderful life. My chest warmed at the thought of Susan being with me through the upcoming months. How bad it would be was anyone's guess—it wasn't sounding so good. But these kinds of thoughtful moments went into forming my plan of how to best tackle the challenge.

I turned off the lights, wound the grandfather clock, and left the office. In my car driving home, I couldn't pay attention to the news on the radio because I kept thinking how grateful I was for knowing how to identify one common source of fear and impairment in a situation like I was in: depression. In my report and progress note writing, I would always refer to the clinical diagnosis with a capital "D" and the colloquial, informal label with a lowercase "d." Many times a day I helped patients see the differences between understandable worry, grief, or "depression" and "Depression." Sadness was not necessarily Depression (with a capital "D"); in fact, it was a normal and healthy emotion that was to be honored and allowed to flow in a sad situation. God gave us tears to wash out our sorrow.

Since I knew the difference, I was equipped to be on the lookout, and so was Susan. After all, depression had been cited as one of the side effects of androgen blockade. I didn't know whether that meant "depression" or "Depression," but in any case, I was already monitoring my mood, along with behaviors like my use of food and drink, work hours, exercise, and regularity of meditation, to name a few. Thankfully, neither of us became Depressed or even depressed.

In my case, if I were to look inward to keep track of my

coping, I certainly knew what to look for. But how many didn't? At the first feelings of heartache or the first flow of tears, many jump to the frightening conclusion of depression and ask for a prescription.

******

In fact, as I thought about the subject, I recalled how two hours earlier I'd been discussing just this topic with Sarah, a young mother of two who had just lost her own mother and whose husband was drinking excessively every day. We walked through the distinction between feeling understandably sad and upset and being depressed. For her, confusion had led her to jump to the frightening conclusion that she was depressed; in fact, she had convinced her primary doctor to prescribe an antidepressant. When that medicine and a second one failed, she came to me for consultation.

I explained to Sarah that Depression is far deeper than unhappiness, and more relentless and corrosive than grief or disappointment. It is a clinical condition that makes one feel sick...heartsick. It can kill. I was probably sounding like a lecturer, but I pointed out that clinical depression's suicide rate is estimated at about 10 to 15 percent among chronic sufferers. Snags become monumental impositions; life loses meaning, and you lose your juice; sleep, appetite, energy, concentration, and libido are disturbed on an everyday basis—nothing is much fun anymore. Humor dies; everything is a chore nearly every day.

She hadn't glazed over but had hung onto every word and then happily shook her head in negation. That hadn't been her situation.

"Patients describe depression as 'firing on half my cylinders,' 'walking knee-deep in mud,' 'having a foggy brain,' or 'being in a black hole,'" I told her.

"That's not me, Doctor. I guess I'm unhappy, then."

That conversation again brought to mind the common fears and confusion about sad feelings. Since I and everyone else at one time or another go through such emotions, it's important to know these distinctions, which is why I talk about them with patients many times a day. Otherwise, fearing being overwhelmed will lead a person to suppress those fears; then the fears go underground without reality testing, creating time bombs, especially in those who have had prior bona fide depression. That's why I kept track of myself each day, though I had never been cursed with depression before. It turned out that I never developed more than understandable worry. For those who had been in a dark place before, many believed that they just couldn't go into another black hole, so they tried to forestall it by denial of ordinary sadness. This comes out in many ways, Tom's rage being just one example.

Another reason I've always made such a point of this ability to look inside at sadness is that it then can be honored, rather than feared, since the universal emotion is part of life's palette. In that light, the pitfall of denial can be avoided. That had not been a problem for me or Susan so far, and I didn't really fear that it would become one. Nonetheless, I would keep a heads-up for it as well as anything else that might cause potential complications.

******

Now, at the end of the second week post-diagnosis, it was time to review my choices. Susan and I had finished our daily end-of-day visit in the living room, our time to share, chat, joke, and plug in. We had a bite to eat, but instead of turning on the news, I excused myself.

"Sweetie, for a change, I need a bit of time to think. Jeez, that's all I'm doing these days. I'm trying to get a clear game plan for what to do and what not to do with my emotions as I go through this. I know it may sound like head-tripping, but it's not. Maybe repeating it to myself helps me to feel like I have a good grip. Anyway, see you in a little while. I'll just be out there on the deck."

"No problem, sweetheart. Just don't obsess. You know what to do already."

With that I smiled and exited through the double French doors out to the deck. Another moonlit night, only now, in the second week, it was a partial moon. I walked to my favorite soft chair and fell into it. Immediately I cleared my head and began to reflect. More directly, I began some conscious work—anticipating and deciding.

I had to choose between "doing damage control" for survival and "squeezing every drop of being alive" for however long I had. And the reports lately had been indicating that I might have some decent chances for years more.

On the one hand, there was the choice I was never going to make--that of just trying to survive and nothing more, a decision based in cynical demoralization captured in the not-so-funny poster: "Life sucks and then you die." I've known so many who have taken this route. Indeed, I've spent my days with many patients who were trying to make sense out of what seems like a senseless world. Often patients would come to me when a personal cataclysm had opened all their old wounds, creating a load that was far too crushing for them. At such times, those survivors hid from themselves, and not going under was their priority. To hell with learning and growing, they would say, and forget plans and expectations; just get through each day. They just needed to tread water, their only goal being that of staying afloat. In effect, their bad habits had taken over. Survival had become more than crisis intervention—it had become a lifestyle and a mind-set.

I would explain to them that when a crisis hit, there certainly was a legitimate need for immediate survival, which would mean holding onto whatever control they could in an uncontrollable situation, no matter what the price, especially if life and limb were at stake. Run, hide, strike back, narrow mental focus, postpone emotional reactions—whatever it took. But that wasn't a long-term solution; it was only effective in a foxhole. At certain points, survival posture was absolutely necessary. When victims felt shattered and broken, making it through each twenty-four-hour cycle with one foot in front of the other was their single most important job.

I'd done crisis survival on the cancer diagnosis day, but thankfully it had been brief. I followed my own advice about not getting stuck once I'd handled the immediate surviving.

Then came the other choice: living. That's when the fundamental challenge would present itself—daring to hope. Hope would be required to open up my mind to want, to need, to feel. Hope would open my spirit to believe, to have faith, to find meaning and purpose. But if I wouldn't dare to hope, I would shut down my heart and soul; I wouldn't be able to allow myself to care, let alone love; I would feel no passion, no awe, no joy; and I would experience no heartache because there would be nothing to be let down about. There would be just a lifeless existence until I keeled over.

Screw that. No way am I going to walk a desert or live in a closet just to avoid the hurts. Hell, that's like saying I would never play any sport because I might get injured. No! Balls to the wall, I take my chances. There's an expression that should go in my archives: "Nothing ventured, nothing gained."

True, my world seemed shattered for a while in the office for those first couple of hours after the cancer call and then on the beach thereafter. But I was able to regroup and stay connected, and I rather quickly grounded myself and stayed open, despite being—to say the least—scared to death. Thank God, I didn't stay in the foxhole.

Since this topic of morale came up for virtually any patient contending with ongoing adversity, I've heard many times that even a simple act of hope could seem dangerous. One person might say, "I can't get my hopes up. I can't take one more letdown." Some have even burdened themselves with an accommodation to sorrow, feeling some comfort from its predictability and imagined controllability. Those survivors described having reached a point of knowing what will happen the next day and the next, saying, "It may be lousy, but it's what I know." Things seemed to them to be better than they were during the assault. I always felt sad for such wounded people and grateful that my emotional baggage had never impaired me like that.

I would discuss with them that the concept of survival has two very different meanings. One, acute survival, is both appropriate and necessary in order to put out the fire. The second, long-term or lifestyle survival, is not so good because it means hiding from life, risking little. The latter one—the dysfunctional survival—means damage control by brainwashing themselves into believing that they had stopped hoping or wanting much. All that had been easy enough to preach, but I had seen firsthand how hard it was for them to switch from immediate lifesaving action to open hope.

Countless songs, poems, and novels have made the

157

point for centuries about taking a chance on life. And everyone has always known that doing so requires morale, juiced by a faith in overall beneficence regardless of doctrine. I wasn't coming up with any novel ideas or insights, but I did promise myself that I would not retreat into mere survival. I always had lived by that promise, and after cancer I wrote the promise in stone.

******

I paused a moment to stand up and stretch, meandering around the deck in continued meditation. I sure as hell was speaking from experience through the years—and especially last week. How else could I have stayed on my game if not by faith in myself, my love, my God, and the medical treatments? With a mixture of gratitude for my gifts and sadness for those souls in hiding, I sat back down in the same comfortable wicker armchair.

A few more thoughts on the central role of faith in my psychology: It has extended beyond positive attitude or self-confidence, and it has been far stronger and more sustaining than a pep talk from a loved one, though that has always helped; rather, I was thinking of faith that has served as my foundation for courage and adventure. It has been the juice that helped me give my best effort. I'd come to think of it as arising from the deepest parts of me to connect me with my sense of the Divine, transcending any mess I might have currently been in. I didn't care if it was called life, or fate, or the Universe, or Spirit, or whatever (Alcoholics Anonymous, or AA, calls it the Higher Power). What I hadn't realized until the day of "The Walk" was that all of those beliefs were not alone down in there. Embarrassing as it was to admit, there were some beliefs that had been out of my awareness, hanging around from my having been a good little boy. Those were the ones that had kept me naïve, believing that being good enough would bring me what I prayed for. Of course, in the interest of Sutton's Law, such innocence had to go. It had nearly killed me.

So there's the value in going over this yet again this evening: Only with such a grown-up grounding can I dare to hope plausibly rather than fancifully. And only with that kind of realistic hope could I give meaning and action to my goals and dreams—like staying alive. A child's magical fantasies won't do it. But with positive belief or grace, I should be able to bounce back and have the will to avoid staying in the foxhole, hiding. We'll see, won't we?

In effect, on the beach during The Walk, I took a leap of faith, especially in my capacity to trust both Susan and God. I had to believe that if I showed up, so would love. Happily for me, God gave me a *nudge*. There was one more concept that I really wanted to nail down for myself. It's the same one I talk about all day long with my patients, but now it was my turn to get it right. The Rule of Holes: Knowing what to do to be emotionally effective is only part of the equation; the other part is knowing what *not* to do.

Hell, I spend all day helping people see how they're shooting themselves in the foot. Well, I've had my own version of that, especially with my crazy naiveté that I didn't need to bother with regular medical care. After all, a good boy like me wouldn't come to harm. I flushed a bit with embarrassment at the mere acknowledgment.

The Rule of Holes is right up there with the Serenity Prayer, the Golden Rule, and Sutton's Law. This one says, "When you're in a hole, don't dig." Those have been fundamental principles for my coping through the years, and they were clearly at work during my cancer plan. I had trouble enough, so I certainly wanted to be sure that I didn't make it worse. In my game plan, I had to be heads-up and deal with two things: bad habits and acts of nature. My bad habits were the everyday things I did that would make any hole deeper; acts of nature were those obstacles or catastrophes that I, like anyone, simply couldn't foresee. And in my case, I even knew many of the screwballs, curves, changeups, and sinkers, but as I've said often, what I didn't expect was the beanball.

I've been aware for years that even the mature among us have dug the hole deeper with sulks, pouts, rage, and cynicism. Sometimes those have been okay as temporary hiding places, especially if the time-out is spent to regroup, but if chronic, such dysfunctions just compound the crisis. For example, how many alcoholics have I known who, during a time of difficulties, fell off the wagon? Or what about the obese person who kept a weight problem at bay but then suddenly dived into comfort foods? There are those who have gone on shopping binges. I smiled as I recalled hundreds of workaholics who, when disaster was near, made the office into a home—they even brought in sheets and a pillow. And there was the common tendency in moments of crisis to withdraw from loved ones and friends. Of course I could relate in some measure to all of them. Maybe I dug my holes with a shovel rather than a backhoe, but I've moved my share of dirt. But at such times I've known enough to pay close attention to signals from family, friends, and colleagues. Often the first sign had come with the realization that people were making more room for me, staying out of my way. My version of digging the hole deeper has usually been to become quiet and uncommunicative. Others often have seen that fallout sooner than I, so I would ask what they were seeing, making sure I was ready to listen to their answers. That was certainly the case with Susan, who helped keep me honest from the first day of this odyssey. I knew that rejecting feedback out of hand could levy a stiff price—besides, that would be plain dumb. If Susan or anyone took the chance to point out something unattractive or dysfunctional, what else could it be but an act of caring? By definition, then, any feedback from a trusted person deserved immediate open-minded attention.

I knew enough to watch out for overeating or extra glasses of wine. Weight gain is a common, even unavoidable, side effect of androgen blockade for prostate cancer. I already had extra pounds; I didn't need more.

I also made ready for another common way to get sidetracked—by allowing disillusionment and disappointment to turn into cynicism and anger at God. What would follow would be a loss of purpose and meaning, what people called being "Godforsaken." I thought I was ready for that one, but it turned out that on the beach it was the beanball I wasn't looking for. There I was, a hip and seasoned psychiatrist, having his little boy tantrum of being left in the lurch. Thankfully I recognized it for what it was, allowed it to run a brief but robust course, and then settled down to recognize the Great Mystery. I knew enough to let it flow and that the dust would settle properly. Of course, it didn't hurt to have Susan waiting for me five miles down the road.

I've known many guilt-ridden persons who have had a very different reaction, seeing the suffering as punishment for past sins, and that interpretation allowed them to see the burden as inevitable and justified. Tom had moments like that. I didn't concern myself with that one; in fact, I went to the opposite extreme of outrage and objection.

Then there was the possibility of the victim response, your basic cavernous hole with bulldozers digging 24/7. Here a yoked and plodding "mule" pulls an unfairly heavy cartload of troubles as he or she wallows in self-pity and self-righteousness. This "mule" may not ask for the troubles out loud but somehow stops the cart every time some heavy burden is nearby and ready for loading. If there are no burdens handy, such a person usually isn't above going down side roads looking for one. Some of the more aware of these patients tease themselves about having pity parties. As I've known for years, my father had become the "mule." Though I had put most of that behind me, there was still a hint of it in my own reactions, so I definitely needed to keep a heads-up to avoid taking up a shovel.

******

A good illustration of the mule myth can be seen in the case of Mrs. W. She came to me for consultation for her fifth depression. Depressions often have physical manifestations, and her downward slide had come along with acute back pain. Barely forty years old, Mrs. W had a litany of woes, which had drained away whatever joy she might have had and rendered her life a shambles. Her most recent hardships took shape in the form of a sprained back. Mrs. W was a nurse's aide, and she had received the injury while lifting an enormous patient out of a wheelchair.

Her workup hadn't indicated any need for surgery, so her doctors recommended a course of physical therapy and mild pain medicine. Physically this made sense, but Mrs. W's primary long-range problem didn't lie in her back. It was when she started talking suicide that her physical therapist hastily guided her to me.

Mrs. W's presentation of her past and present crises was so well organized and clear that her recitations of them had the feel of long hours of rehearsal. I didn't think that she'd rehearsed these lists of troubles for my benefit; rather, I assumed that she had gone over them again and again for herself, possibly speaking them out loud until they became a kind of mantra.

The lists were long, and she seldom had a shortage of new items to add to them. Events seemed to concoct themselves purely for the purpose of furthering her misery. The causes and people involved were different every time, but the result was always the same: her downfall. She felt little or no responsibility for her choices and seemed to relish the telling, as if her suffering were a unique source of virtue. I knew that this wasn't the best way for her to make the most of a bad situation.

Accompanying the ill fortune and persecution was always physical pain. Her body had become a vessel holding the pains of her trials and tribulations. Arthritis, earaches, respiratory infections, and multiple orthopedic injuries from car wrecks and falls made up much of the list.

Her difficulties had begun in childhood with sexual abuse. Following this came teenage assaults, date rape, early marriage to a total loser, and three car wrecks. Along with these came two more husbands and five terribly troubled children, not to mention her depressions. As I've noted, her depressions had their physical effects, yet she refused to follow a steady course of medication. Mrs. W trudged from one heartache to the next, knowing disaster would come but never seeing her prophecies as self-fulfilling.

Where could we begin? The events were real, as were the depressions. Her sprained back was no more faked than a badly broken limb, yet as she walked into each calamity, eyes open, she could only perceive her injuries as coming from outside of her. She'd resigned herself to powerlessness, so each day was no more than an exercise in damage control.

I didn't question the real consequences of her sorrow,

shame, and impotence. I gave them validation, but I did not accept them as inevitable. That was the crack in her mythology through which some light might peek—her possibility for hope lay in her responses themselves; that is, she hurt because life mattered. She wanted to stop suffering for her own interests of comfort. In effect, we began to talk the language of wanting and needing and started to build a mind-set of looking for relief and comfort, of improving her lot. She shifted from a complaining resignation to pain to an expectation of relief.

It happened gradually. Slowly, our shift toward the possible gave her an awareness of autonomous, active choices. She learned that she could feel all emotions, not just those rooted in self-pity, and regained the capacity to have just enough hope to take a different look. As she started to master the terrifying feelings of outrage, fear, and shame, she didn't have to hide from them in the victim role. She started to get unstuck.

This was a process of rebuilding her morale. The action was not in what the medical events themselves were but rather in how she saw them and put them into her life picture. Slowly, as a consequence of daring to walk through her journey with me, she was able to realize that her reactions indicated that she cared, that she mattered. Otherwise, why would she complain? The internal changes were not confined to increased personal insight or understanding; they also arose as a natural part of experiencing the journey. As I often reassured her, especially when she was confused at apparent complexity, "Not to worry, the healing is in the feeling. Let's just keep walking. Your heart naturally wants to heal. We're giving it a chance with some loving honesty—as if it were fresh air."

In Mrs. W, this growth to openness was necessary so that emotional and spiritual healing could begin. She found the courage and confidence to open a route to her accumulated emotional turmoil hidden in the basement, so to speak. She needed her truth for empowerment; then she could begin emerging from hiding in survival's closet. She began to feel in charge, stopped seeing herself as living under a dark cloud, and became proactive.

Mrs. W was a good example of emotional responses that are amplified or even determined by the accumulated echoes of past hurts. Victim mythology was repeatedly reinforced by her perceptions, which were locked in place by feelings that she had frozen in order to hide. She couldn't hide if the emotional pain burst forth honestly and if she allowed herself to see, so it required blinders and brainwashing. Each trauma was a reliving of past tumults, magnifying the depth of any given hurt. Each one echoed out of the darkness of the basement, quite out of her awareness as it had been designed to be.

I thought about her in that meditation because her example captured the pathos and impotence of the mule myth. I felt sad for my father and frightened for myself, lest I go anywhere near.

******

"Hey, Sigmund, the special on blues is about to start. Finish up figuring out the universe and your game plan or whatever you call it. Also, the hot tub is heating."

It was a reality check from Susan, bless her. So much for physical and emotional readiness. The cultivation of morale was equally—if not more—important. I vowed not to lose heart or faith.

Chapter 13
The Spiritual Challenge

The Great Mystery offers no assurances, justice, reward, or punishment. Prayer is for courage and help, not for outcomes. Santa Claus works for kids, not for grown-ups.

Our dock reached out thirty feet into the shimmering lagoon. One Sunday, three weeks after the big day, I sat at the far end with legs dangling, relishing the spectacular view to the north, two miles up the placid water. A tropical scene fit for a calendar—I loved this spot for its beauty and isolation. Cormorants dived and resurfaced; mullet swarmed just under the surface, leaving swirls to evidence their activity. Late afternoon was arriving, bringing with it a cooling breeze. The afternoon had been filled with phone calls from well-wishers and with trips to the medical supply store to purchase a urinal that was more substantial than the light plastic ones I had found in the pharmacy the week before. I hoped that I wouldn't need one for as long as I had heard (a year or more), but I wanted to be ready for anything. One guy from Man to Man had spoken of over eighteen months of urinary frequency to the tune of a dozen times a day, and the same for nights.

At least I was dealing with a cancer that potentially could be contained and killed so that I could live. Hope for longer life was plausible, not just quality for whatever little time remained. But what of men who knew their cancer had spread? At that thought, my heart was heavy with sadness for all of them.

Maybe I can beat this. Thank you, God, for the chance.

Energized by my chances, I looked ahead in earnest at the treatments and at the heart and soul challenges. Grabbing the opportunity for a peaceful moment of repose, I settled into thoughts about how I had begun to come to terms on the beach three weeks ago. It had taken cancer to shake me loose and turn my face to the mystery of life. And out there at the end of the dock, I thought about my future, and whether I even had one. I realized that in many ways, the greatest threat wasn't physical. Pain and limitations I could handle in stride, one day at a time, and whatever downtime there would be, well, I would roll with it. But my heart and soul were to be different, especially the latter. The cancer had forced me to admit how fragile life is and how a heartbeat or a phone call can turn it upside down in a flash. Of course I had known all that, but now the shoe was actually on my foot.

Within my physical crisis of life or death was a spiritual crisis of morale or faith. Would I be able to maintain my optimism and confidence? Those days I often asked myself whether I could continue to find purpose right up to the end, if this became an ending.

Will I die well if it comes to that?

I chucked a small shell out into the water and watched the circles it generated. From the center of impact spread ever-widening reverberations.

No...no dorky metaphors, Bobby. Stay on track here.

I shrugged and took a deep breath, exhaling slowly. I sure had lost my innocence. For one thing, I hadn't really been living with the daily recognition that I could die, actually dry up and blow away. Finito. Caput. Somehow, no matter how much I had seen and how many deaths I had attended in medicine, I'd kept my healthy denial. Of course I had to—or I never would have come out to play. But cancer blew that cover. I scuffed the water's surface below me, and my reflection disintegrated into a kaleidoscope. It had become real clear that, like it or not, faith was not about asking for detailed outcomes.

True, I had started to find renewed love and faith on the beach three weeks earlier.

Maybe it was because the beach was Susan's place and she had always brought out the best in me. Or maybe it was that God-given sunset. Or maybe it was just the time in my journey to grow up. Whatever...

I recalled how I began to talk to God. At first it was a tantrum that I knew had to come out. It was part of getting to my truth. But then it became more of a conversation. Most of us call that prayer.

With the bitterness of disillusionment now gone, I could look back on that fast-track beach passage and feel grateful for coming to peace with the fact that the best I could do was to ask God for support.

Of course, I'd wanted answers and a cure. Who wouldn't? But, Bobby Boy, gone are the days of asking for Buffalo Bob's brown and white pony in the backyard tomorrow morning.

169

So I started to look inside more than ever to find loving connections, my own gifts, and God's support. That was the route to my resilience, not being on my knees begging and waiting passively for God to do His magic for me.

I shifted my seating position because my butt was starting to hurt as I sat on the wooden planks. With that distraction relieved, I thought about those acquaintances or patients who had reacted to their traumas by turning away from the truth and trying to burrow into some kind of a womb for protection. "Out of sight, out of mind" became their motto. "OK, you have cancer. Get over it."

Hell, there must have been dozens of old-fashioned platitudes or homilies for grandma's advice. None of them work except in the midst of a gunfight during which you just dive for cover and shoot back while hoping for the best.

Others reacted with bluster, telling the world—and themselves—that they could easily beat anything or anyone. "OK, something's wrong, but I'll kick its ass." That one reminded me of being eight years old and walking through a haunted house, whistling in the dark as I peed my pants. Others will stuff feelings by saying, "Don't cry over spilt milk."

Those cliché recipes were long on denial, I grinned, and denial in the long run can be fatal. Only truth worked.

So I dangled, stared, made little waves, and even chucked another shell out into the water. As expected, the concentric circles reappeared.

******

I wanted to imprint the lessons in my brain. I wanted to live what I knew, like how essential it has been, and would continue to be, to stay open and to avoid bamboozling. Specifically, that meant no Superdoc nonsense and no childish tantrum. As for squaring my relationship with God, I had to hold to the belief that His larger plan would work out for the good, no matter how obscure that seemed at any given moment, even if it included death. And it sure was obscure.

I got up, stretched, and walked a bit on the dock to loosen up my buttocks, which by that time had started to ache. Of course the swollen killer in my prostate could have been contributing.

Why not? It was trying to screw up everything else.

I looked underneath our overturned wooden boat in search of a seat cushion. A few roaches and a small snake later, I extracted the cushion and placed it at my spot at dock's end. I lowered myself back down into position.

Ahhh...that feels better.

The instructive value in my again taking stock was to remind myself of how unspectacular or ordinary I had been in my movement through life's ups and downs. I'd coped pretty much like most anyone. But especially helpful in my many recent introspections had been learning more about how I had handled the blindside hit from which I was still reeling. The greatest insight had come from the opportunity to see, once again, the way I unknowingly had set myself up for a crisis. Admittedly, I wasn't talking about causing my cancer, though perhaps a more alkaline diet through the years might have helped with prevention. Instead, I was referring to the way my immature mythology had rendered me naïve or unaware of some aspects of the crisis that took me by surprise. The spiritual tantrum that Santa Claus screwed up and left walnuts and razor blades in my stocking instead of a new train set...well, that was a problem. The star nonsense, it had turned out, had been my Achilles' heel.

I decided to leave it at that, especially since my

stomach was growling in hunger. Maybe I could grab a bite of that lily over there on my way in for a salad.

Oh, yeah, it beats the box.

******

Over three weeks had passed since the big hit of the cancer call. I was keeping to my plan of morning workouts and full workdays, and my clinical work was more empathic than ever as I drew from my own reactions. Susan and I had just had our daily visit and pleasant meal on the deck. Then I wanted to walk and think. I sure was doing a lot of that those days. But why not? This was, after all, the biggest crisis I'd ever faced. I needed to be proactive—and I was. I took any chance I could to reflect, take inventory, make corrections, and plan, so I headed out for a walk down the sidewalk to Turtle Beach to our south.

I liked strolling Midnight Pass Road at dusk. It was a good time to collect my thoughts and brainstorm; it was also a time to reflect backwards weeks, months, or years. I liked putting together the story, making sense out of patterns or developmental sequences. The clearer picture was like a map, and a detailed map meant direction, a route with few blind alleys or surprises. So I took the opportunity that cool fall evening for an overview of the past few decades, especially the parts about some of my heart and soul growth, as the air was starting to cool down and the traffic had let up for the day.

Despite excellent mechanics-driven education and clinical training, through my early years of doctoring I'd remained, as both person and physician, connected heart to heart with my patients. I just didn't label it as anything more than kind and sensitive back then; like in all the rest of medicine, I didn't regard that as a so-called spiritual dimension. After all, I'd been trained to be the hardworking hotshot at a time when such thinking was not part of medical education. My caring way was just another natural capacity. I didn't think much about it because it was just the way I was. Twenty-five years ago, I could not have made the distinction. As far as I knew, I was genuinely kind and caring; it all seemed to work. Thereafter, my success in practice spoke for itself, and patients often directly expressed their gratitude.

My early religious experience was Roman Catholic on account of my father; my mother was Episcopalian. But orthodoxy never caught me, so religious practice didn't become important in my early growth. Morality and ethics, however, were always fundamental in our family. In any event, by the time I was in medical school witnessing the miracles of life and biology, I began to become keenly interested in spirituality and the big picture, but only in privacy. From there, I wrestled with the universal task of contending with life's obvious paradoxes and frailties. How could I avoid the issues, what with my attending to those dealing with pain, healing, madness, and death?

In those days of being a young physician, my peers and I just assumed that kindness, politeness, and professional dignity were parts of the highly valued cultural image of the physician, simply the right way to be, which was called "bedside manner." With me these traits were natural and became my basis for good doctoring without much self-conscious thought. I never named them as spiritual and certainly not metaphysical. No one would have credited these gifts with any power to heal. I sure didn't, except in a general sense of good practice. At that early stage, I knew nothing about the healing of faith and positive intention, with such ideas being ridiculed as mere "placebo response."

I picked up the pace a bit, trying to stretch my legs. I noted that in recent years I had read and learned of energy healing and had been enthused. I found validation from my mother's example as well as growing social acceptance of the mind/body connection. I'd attended seminars on spirituality and medicine and had started to read the compelling research on healing touch and distant healing. And to boot, ideas and practices from this powerful but "fuzzy" dimension were becoming increasingly valid in the public's mind. I had even consulted several metaphysical adepts, each of whom underscored my intuitive gifts and proclivity to the spiritual.

As time went on into the 1980s, I felt grateful that as the views of society changed, I was able to openly express this aspect of myself in the professional realm. I even smiled quietly as I recalled how more and more of my shoptalk with my father had involved psychological issues. Now and then, I snuck in spiritual ideas such as morale supported by meditation. I began with cautious exploration and in time was emboldened to go further. But there were limits. My few attempts to speak of distant healing remained in the relatively safe venues of orthodox Catholic prayer and/or miracles. Dad understood and operated within the commonsense versions of such metaphysical concepts; nonetheless, he was in the dark about any contemporary thinking beyond his conservative views, so I was just happy to take it as far as he could go, which was a lot further than thirty years earlier.

I couldn't resist musing that if only my father had been born a century earlier, he would have learned medicine in a world where physicians were healers, teachers, ministers, and parent figures, all in one. But, understandably, he didn't identify with those historical values. He'd gone through his own phase as a young upwardly mobile immigrant son in the new scientific age. The mind was personal and informal, and religion was left to the church. He was a product of his time. Who wasn't?

So only some of our talks were congenial; others were disappointing. Dad respected my point of view but remained entrenched in his way of thinking. To his great credit, he always admitted being influenced by the post–World War II decades. For him, medical healing was aimed at the body, while the soul was separate.

Although I'm sure he had high hopes when I did an internal medicine internship at Yale where he was an attending physician, he never chastised me for not following his path, nor did he ever insult my choice of the emerging field of psychiatry, about which he'd known next to nothing. He always had the grace to say little of it one way or the other.

His loving loyalty to me went so far as to prompt him to send me articles on psychosomatic medicine. He stretched his envelope that far, but no further. Nonetheless, his pride and regard for my overall success were unshakable, even to the point of turning to me for personal advice in his last years. Perhaps the closing of the circle indicated some resolution of the myths.

Medical school gave way to residency, specialty training, and then my own practice. My life went from busy to busier, and as I rolled through the blur of activity in my thirties and forties, I was still able to learn new things. I didn't completely neglect the metaphysical; it was simply a matter of keeping it under wraps. Nonetheless, I began to see its effects in my professional life. Many lessons that I'd never learned in formal training came from my daily psychiatric practice. I've been continually privileged to hear my patients' stories of triumph and tragedy, and through the decades, their morale has never ceased to interest and amaze me.

Their emotional and spiritual struggles certainly have helped me to make sense of this fragile life, especially lately as I've come to face my own mortality.

As the years passed in clinical work, I had to contend with my impotence in the face of infinitely complex human nature and biology. Hearing so many stories of undeserved trauma was tough enough, but my own limitations kept coming to the fore.

How could I help my patients change their behavior and do things constructively? Could I help them find meaning in the face of a horrid loss or tragedy...without empty platitudes? What should I say, for example, to a mother wracked with grief over her child's suicide? Was there really something helpful in lending an ear or feeling badly, or was that just futile posturing? Could I really touch hearts and souls to promote their healing?

Those questions often left me frustrated. I kept looking at people and trying to figure out how to "fix" them. Early on in my growth as a physician I didn't recognize the restorative value of lending my heart to a suffering patient.

Illness and trauma were never just or fair, making them all the more puzzling, yet thankfully I never became cynical or pessimistic. My faith and even my mythology helped there. I was indefatigable; I never gave up my optimistic outlook. But early on, this was a function more of my mythology than of deep humility and spiritual faith—never mind wisdom.

Man, can I now see the setup for a loss of innocence when the wake-up call sounded. No wonder it hit me like it did.

I heard the tinkle of a bicycle bell coming from behind me on the sidewalk just in time to move out of the way. An elderly man smiled and excused himself politely as he nearly took me out. I must have been so absorbed in thought that I hadn't heard him coming. Soon my brief adrenaline rush settled down as I resumed my walk. I focused my breath and went back into reverie. The house wasn't far ahead down the street, and I could just make out the white mailbox with the white lattice base.

How odd that central to my outlook has always been a conviction that I must be destined to give care in the face of fragility and loss of control over one's mind. Why else go into this field? My patients' bewilderment and disillusionment have only steeled my resolve to delve further into the Great Mystery, though early on I would have called it the fascinating unknown.

My faith remained intact in recent years even as the Great Mystery became more apparent, though it hadn't been personally tested until I got cancer.

Whether I looked for it or not, I know divine guidance has been there.

So after all was done, I didn't have to rely completely on my star myth's belief in competence. At both personal and professional levels, I'd been spiritually plugged into the universe for more than a decade, fueling my own grounding and peace. It also gave me a view of life captured in—among other things—the Serenity Prayer. In short, my capacity steadily grew for empathizing with my patients' courageous struggles to uphold their morale; in fact, it deepened without my conscious effort. How lucky was I? My patients' personal growth showed me firsthand that demoralized helplessness can be transformed into spirited empowerment. They taught me more than I'd ever known about the possibilities of rising above the fragilities of life to see its wonders.

I thank every one of you.

I recalled talking with a patient, Justine, just recently,

making the point about how crises, along with our biology, give shape to the landscape of our lives. We talked about her chronic pulmonary disease and her divorce, illustrating how none of that kind of trauma was ever deserved and, thankfully, how suffering and despair were not necessarily the only options that one has to look forward to. As easy as it was to say rather than do, and without minimizing her legitimate suffering, we both agreed that the impact of her situation was always what she made it to be. Therein lay her hope. In similar situations I've witnessed incredible tenacity and courage, even when old wounds open, compounding the challenge. She and many other patients showed me morale in action. We also agreed that humor and irony were two of the best tools for making headway through a morass (she liked to laugh, even though it further taxed her breathing).

I was nearly at the entrance to our driveway. I rounded the entrance column in the front garden and started down the shell drive. Just like on diagnosis day, when I heard the shells crunch under the car wheels, I heard them answer again that evening under my feet. Dusk was melting into early darkness, so all the house lights lit up the white clapboard exterior and the second-story deck railings, above which soared the high peaked roofline. Inside, the brass chandelier shone through the second-floor-deck French doors as it hung majestically from the high cathedral ceiling over the entrance atrium. Was I ever lucky to have such a beautiful retreat! I savored the moment like it might be one of my last, as I was wont to do these days. This time my approach wasn't frantic or as pained because I was centered on my task of handling my cancer workup and treatments, along with their emotional and spiritual impact. I was developing my three-point approach of physical, emotional, and spiritual readiness.

******

I imposed a bit on Susan to once again hear more about my story, this time with the added insights from my cancer crisis.

She's already heard all that, my man. How many times are you going to impose on her patience for repetition? Yes…there's always a new twist, so let's hope she's okay with more. This better not be just obsessing.

I was on a roll that evening, so I entered the house and climbed the winding stairs with a springy step, and we greeted each other.

"Hey, sweetheart, where have you been the past half hour? I went to check outside to see if you had keeled over into the bushes. They were clear, so I guessed that you went for that walk."

"Yes, my dear, I did. And thanks for the death watch. I walked down to the park and back. I meditated as I went, so I'm into it. Do you have a few minutes to indulge me to talk out loud so I can continue?"

"Of course. Let's sit out on the deck"

We made ourselves comfortable in the white wicker chairs with the soft tufted seats. It turned out that, as always, she willingly spent all the time I needed that evening, even listening seriously. But if I got a bit too heavy, and certainly if I started to wax eloquent, she would nail it, rolling her eyes or smirking good-naturedly.

"As you know from probably too many conversations lately, I'm trying to learn what I can from this intruder. What I'm thinking about this evening is how I matured, or failed to, as a man and a doctor in terms of emotional and spiritual depth. In other words, why I was so thrown for a loop and outraged at getting cancer? Moi?! Remember D-day and what I went through on the beach? Those issues?"

179

"No problem. Shoot."

"Well, I'm thinking that even as I developed a more holistic approach in medicine through the 1970s and 1980s, I didn't realize it, but underneath all the broad-mindedness I was still just a little grownup star. I hate to suggest it, but maybe my sense of destiny was so ingrained that my on-the-job learning and success only fostered a naïve sense of potency. In the trade we call it omnipotence."

"Yes, Sigmund. I know. Go ahead."

"Okay, right. Look…if this is an imposition…"

"Oh come on, Bob. Of course I want to hear it. Just don't get precious on me. You know I'm kidding. Please continue."

Her tone softened, inviting warmth, and I went ahead and reviewed with her how, over the past decade or so, I'd developed a much better appreciation of the role real-life obstacles and challenges have in complicating a person's biology. And although I'd made morale and hope a greater part of my clinical work, I'd apparently not developed these fully enough into an integrated outlook. I told her that, in retrospect, D day had shown me that some of my maturity was merely the trapping of my Superdoc business, underneath which lay remnants of adolescent omnipotence.

"Honey, that shit's hard to admit. I wasn't as free from my past as I'd thought."

"Tell me something we don't know."

"Yeah. But I need to do this again out loud. Just a minute more."

Despite her glazed-over expression, emphasized for effect, she nodded, "Go ahead," and sighed dramatically in feigned boredom.

"Had I remained stuck in that stage, my response to cancer would have been quite limited. I would have told the boy to shut up, pushed him back into my unconscious, and taken care of the immediate medical business. But I would've missed the wake-up call for growth—in short, I would've blown it. Fortunately I didn't."

"Thanks, sweetie, that takes us to a good stopping point. You already know all this. You did respond positively. Enough, already. You don't need to beat it to death...no pun intended. Can I get you some fruit? A late dessert would be nice."

******

Later that night, still savoring the non-alkaline indulgence, I sat in the dark on the deck overlooking the lagoon. Shimmering, the big moon danced over the water, which was slightly perturbed by a gentle breeze, and the warm glow from inside the house fell onto the deck all around me. I settled back into the wicker armchair, which by that time had become a therapy chair, adjusted the pillows, and gazed out at the dark silhouette of palms across the water. A couple of deep breaths and I was centered.

For reasons that weren't immediately apparent, this train of thought about spirituality led me again to my mother. For over a decade, she had been caught in the slow suffering of dementia, and forgetfulness had magnified into increasingly irrational behavior. By the time I moved to Florida, she needed to move with me. Her devolving clinical status required an intensively supportive group living arrangement, followed thereafter by a nursing home life that most people would describe as "vegetative." At that point she required round-the-clock care. Because I knew this was likely coming, I placed her in a nearby facility so that I could visit her even when she reached the point of not recognizing me. In fact, in her last years she knew no one; she hardly uttered a word, lying bedridden in the fetal position. In many ways, the woman who had been my mother was gone, but her body was so free of formal disease (except for dementia) that she lasted far longer than most. As her son, I bore witness to this dying process, with all its spiritual and emotional difficulties.

Tears welled, and my heart was wrenched and heavy as I pressed on. Anyone who has dealt with lingering death knows this sadness, but for me there was also the challenge of trying to understand. I wondered about the usual things—issues that arise when seeing someone, our own flesh and blood, who seemed to be both there and gone.

Is Mom gone in spirit? What did her physical presence here in this room mean? What about an afterlife?

It began to occur to me that there might be a purpose even in this apparently tragic manifestation of her. Since then, the idea has grown within me that my mother was still there, in spirit as well as failing body, using her seemingly failed state to challenge me. In her conscious years on this earth, she had watched and encouraged the process of my becoming the star. She'd given me her unquestioning love, but I'm sure she had also hoped I would grow beyond that to see something of what her own life was about.

I'd returned her love with my own but always had reserved the real respect and honor for my father's profession. Through my youth and on into my early practice, I'd subscribed to his intellectualized way of seeing the world. Admiring and imitating Dad, I debunked much of Mom's way of thinking as nonsense. I really felt sad recalling this and wiped away a tear.

Easy, Bobby...that's the way it was. The entire journey was necessary, from foolish naiveté to maturity. You had to miss out on her, but her gifts are now all the more precious for it. That's what growth is about. Just be grateful you

*kept moving on and growing. Today you embrace Mom's
benefactions as much as you do Dad's. I could vividly
imagine her lying there, giving no clear idea of whether she
was in this world or the next.*

Meanwhile, in the years since her illness had taken
over, I'd found myself entertaining more and more of my
intuition. At the end, I was faced with a body whose
clinical meaning was little more than a pulse rate and the
throbbing of a few involuntary muscles, yet it was she.
Could she be daring me to come to grips with the spiritual
and metaphysical? Was I ready to deal with these issues in
my mother's lingering death?

At that moment of tragedy, it was hard to tell and I
couldn't even articulate the whole question. I had come a
long way, but had I really seen the mind/body/spirit
connection in her effort? I thought I had, in terms of my
work; I also gave evidence of coming to grips with it in my
new loving relationship with my true soul mate. There were
even strong indications of my progress in my friendships
and in my work with patients.

But there was my mother's body, curled into the shape
of a fetus in the womb. As death slowly engulfed her, I
watched, thought, felt,...and struggled for answers.

I know now that in her slow death my mother gave me
the ultimate gift: the chance to face the Great Mystery. I
smiled and my heart lightened. That's why I went out to the
dock that evening, to recognize her gift to me.

My father had also died, but that had been different. His
demise hadn't had that kind of slow drama because he had
died suddenly and unexpectedly of a heart attack at the
wheel of his car, parked in his driveway, and a sheriff had
called to inform me. His death had come in an earlier and
different phase of my life when I'd been a different man,
busily focused on my day-to-day doings.

Each death came at a different phase of my life, separated by fifteen years. I grieved for him in his style, just as I later grieved for Mom in hers. What a difference in access to heart and soul. My good-byes to both were only to their physical selves—inside me, over the years, the best of both of them grew, giving me a mixture of gifts and vulnerabilities.

My sons had been young enough at the time of my father's death in the early 1980s to still need me every day. Each day I'd been working in a practice and a medical establishment that my father had done so much to define. In a way, Dad's sudden death had seemed as nuts and bolts as his view of life and medicine. He had died, I had grieved, grief had passed, and I carried the torch forward. Each had taken its predictable turn.

Regarding my being grateful to Mom for her open-mindedness to pushing the envelope, wouldn't she be proud of my burgeoning interest in complementary medicine? My interest in Eastern medicine began with my practicing acupuncture in the early '70s, but I really started in earnest in the mid-'80s as I investigated vibrational medicine, a field comprising energy-based healing through acupuncture, herbs, oils, and homeopathic flower remedies. My interests also came to include neuromuscular massage, healing touch, Reike, Tua Na, craniosacral massage, and other massage methods. Some became part of both my clinical work and my own self-care.

My own practice of prayer began in traditional Catholic orthodox recitation but had evolved into meditative prayer. I now realize that I've just begun to pray with maturity.

I was so impressed by Herbert Bensen's groundbreaking work—*Relaxation Response*—that I incorporated it into my teaching and clinical practice. It also formed my early meditation practice, along with Qigong, tai chi, and yoga—all disciplines that involve or complement meditation.

In the early 1990s, I learned to practice Qigong, the Chinese practice of energy nourishment and healing, and have practiced this form of meditation daily for over fifteen years. Also I learned tai chi, practicing it for several years in the mid-1990s. To this day, I meditate every day, many times during the day. Some are wonderful trips of up to an hour in a quiet place at home, usually mornings; others are brief conversations or pauses throughout the day.

I've been connected for some time, building up to that over the past decade. I never made much of a fuss about it since it just seemed to have become my way, thinking through personal matters and clinical issues in reflective and active communication. My faith and inner way of being and relating had been growing for ten to fifteen years, setting me up for the big one. Contemplating that explosion gave me a whole new sense of faith and prayer.

For many years, I was trying to find a fitting place for my beliefs within the world of religion and developing my sense of living in spirituality. At the same time, through the 1980s and early 1990s, there arose a growing public interest in spirituality and health. Research began to appear and was reported in serious journals; several books by Gerber, Dossey, and others made metaphysical ideas accessible to those of us without extensive education in the field. My mind was blown: Here was validation to offset my lifelong uneasiness with breeching Dad's mind-set! And there was a marvelous body of literature to enjoy as well as to suggest to my patients.

I studied palliative care and immersed myself in research on distant healing, energy work, and the power of prayer. I wanted to formalize my marriage with the spiritual paradigm in health care, so I became ordained in the Universal Church of the Master, a nondenominational

Christian church focused on direct communication with God's loving energy. I even devoted a room in my office suite as a chartered nondenominational chapel, called Trilogy Chapel. That kicked things up a notch, in the context of a shift in my whole orientation toward mind/body/spirit.

But in retrospect, I could see that the mind/body/spirit connections hadn't quite matured. Not surprisingly, the next in-depth step came from the fluidity of my cancer crisis. In the shake-up I saw a clearer truth.

I sure did.

I nodded as I recalled diagnosis day.

That was some day.

I've performed a few weddings and funeral services as a minister, but I've come to realize that my ministry has counted more in what I have done every day. Mine is 24/7, with no need for a standing structure called a church. My church resides in my offices, in the hospitals and clinics where I practice, and in my home. They've all been sacred places.

For me, medicine is a sacred profession.

As I sat still on the deck, I shifted my scope to a wider angle, a panorama of years since my arrival here. I saw how I've discovered a sense of the sacred suffusing all my relationships—those with friends, family, and strangers. Now, in the short time since my cancer diagnosis, this sacred sense has seemed to be more and more one of awe. I no longer view my relationships from the nuts-and-bolts viewpoint of tit-for-tat responsibilities and loyalties, nor have I seen my work as one of simple goal-directed labor. Responsibility and hard work have remained important elements, of course, but they are enriched by my inner sense of the Great Mystery.

I've had enough for one day. My mind is tired and I've

re-experienced many emotions, but I feel productive. The pieces fit just a bit better, so time to go inside to read something light.

******

Nonetheless, even heading back into the house, images and vignettes about spirituality continued to flood my mind. So I lingered in thought long enough to recall having met with an inquisitive patient, Sally M., a 44-year-old mother of two and a store manager, at the office earlier that day.

"Tell me, Doctor, what is faith anyway? I read the Bible, say my prayers, and behave myself, but I'm not sure you and I are talking about the same thing here."

"Well, maybe not, Sally, but let me explain what it has been to me. You will decide for yourself."

"Good."

"For starters, I've come to realize that my own energy and will have their limits. The Serenity Prayer is one of my rules of life. I've lost a naïve illusion that I had harbored deep down about being some kind of star child who rated divine favors if I just kept being a good boy. I've known for some time that I, like you and everyone, get crashed on from time to time (some people feel like it's all the time). My lumps have forced me to ponder the issue of faith more deeply than I did as a kid when the action was just to believe and accept." I went on to explain that, above all, my wondrous patients had taught me about having morale and bouncing back, and that the critical factor in being resilient and maintaining purpose was faith or connection.

"That's fine, but faith in what? Connection to what?" she asked with her inquisitive tenacity. "Is faith blind? Is it just a 'nice, nice' for little boys and girls? Is it, as some of

187

you psychoanalysts think, just a ploy to defend against worry and uncertainty? Are we talking about merely a psychological defense mechanism?"

"Sally, you always ask the most telling questions. Thank you. No, for me it's neither blind nor protective, and it's more than self-confidence or optimism. I experience it as a transcendental connection. It's a basic ingredient for giving me the juice to make as much as I can out of this life."

I continued by suggesting that faith is not naïve or contrived. It has offered me a way to hold my belief in possibilities and overall goodness despite failure and disappointment. Without it, practicing my personal best would be ridiculously hard. Sally would decide for herself what to make of these issues, but I offered her my ideas for what they were worth.

I took it a step further and asserted that I experienced faith as inspiration and sustenance in the face of life's mystery. It has been the juice that has fed my courage, and with it, I've been able to keep my eye on the big picture when evil seems to be winning; it has allowed me to make sense out of nonsense. I expressed my hope that she, too, would find her own way of making sense out of nonsense, order out of apparent disarray.

"But," I added, "it's not a philosophical posture about the absence of doubt. In fact, it permits doubt. Mature faith is surely not blind."

"Well, you've said what it does for you, but what is it? Where does it come from?"

"Well, Sally, if I could answer that well, I would be a philosopher or theologian. But since I'm neither, I can only say that it is a force, an energy that comes from down deep and from a divine source, and stays firm like a solid base when all else seems to be upside down. It can't be faked or manufactured, and I haven't been able to force it to happen."

With some hesitation about stepping on her religious toes, I ventured further that whereas faith may be defined in Scripture or philosophical writings, it doesn't originate in them, nor does it come from fear. The faith-like feeling that fear inspires is more like granting the demands of an extortionist in return for survival. I didn't rule out the possibility of genuine conversion in the midst of danger, but if these conversions were to be lasting, they must have been based on a greater search for true meaning. I hoped that I wasn't offending her beliefs, but she had asked.

"In fact, I'm reminded of Garrison Keillor's joke on the radio show "Prairie Home Companion" about spirituality or faith versus protocols or orthodoxy. Paraphrased, it goes something like this: 'Just going to church and expecting to become religious is like sitting in the garage and expecting to become a car.'"

I shared that after all was said and done, one day I stopped thinking and analyzing so much, put aside my intellectual teachings, and listened. Experience in the moment seemed truer, more direct, than lots of analysis. I wasn't disparaging psychological thought; I just realized that it went only so far. So I shut up, stopped the mind chatter, and listened, like I'd read in some books. Guess what? Suddenly the awareness sprang forth from God as a free gift. I just had to get out of the way and open up my heart and spirit. It came naturally through a universal connection that I had been cultivating and preparing with meditation practice and that I finally allowed to happen. The operative word is "allowed," not "made" or "determined."

"In a way, Doctor Mignone, you're saying, "Sit down, shut up, tune in, and let the connection happen.'"

189

"Yes, that's it, Sally. At some point you stop trying to control the uncontrollable. As one of my former patients put it, 'You can't push the river.'"

"Thanks, Doctor M. I'll think about all that."

As for me, I was as prepared as I could get myself to take on the Grim Reaper. I'd really had enough for one day.

Chapter 14

Game On

The blow by blow of turning off the gonads, zapping the cancer, and keeping up with my practice, marriage, and personhood. And all the while staring the Grim Reaper in the face.

In late October 2003, treatment began for focal cancer—the game was on. Diagnosis day had been in late August, at the end of the hot Florida summer of 2003. The next couple of weeks had been a time of investigation and not a little soul-searching. I'd learned a lot about myself and about the medical/surgical options. I had a fairly good idea of what would be in store and had prepared as best I could, from urinals and diapers to a psychological/spiritual game plan. During that time, I settled on the course of my two-part treatment: first, temporary chemical castration and external irradiation; second, radioactive seed implants.

My treatment started in late October with radiation

oncology (testosterone blockade) combined with blasting the cancer with external radiation for five weeks, five days a week. The hormone-blocking therapy, Casodex and Proscar, shut down my testosterone system, which would put a lid on the male hormones and starve the cancer. This began the androgen blockade, but I wouldn't begin feeling the side effects until several weeks after that. It was a slow form of temporary chemical castration that was to last four to six months.

For the external radiation, also starting in late October, I arrived at the facility each weekday morning for five weeks at the same time: 7:30 A.M. The wait was short; then I was summoned to the treatment room behind leaded walls and doors. I lay on a movable table on my back, my legs and feet secured in a Styrofoam mold fabricated to hold my body still. I had to be sure to wear the same shoes each time so as not to throw off the settings. The routine was the same and the staff was always friendly.

"Morning, Doctor. You know the drill. Drop your trousers just enough to expose your lower abdomen. Let's do this quick ultrasound to make sure your bladder has enough water in it from those glasses of water we've asked you to drink before coming in... oh yes, it's fine. So just hold still while I slide this table into the machine."

The radiation was delivered via a stereotaxic beam from the big donut-like machine, amazingly accurate and aimed at very specific targets in the prostate gland. Its precision virtually guaranteed little chance of collateral tissue damage, and the treatments were painless. I was warned not to wear out my shoes in mid-treatment, including the three months of follow-up, after the seeding in December. Once again, the devil was in the details.

I rode the slow sliding table into a big fat donut, which moved on its axis upon command from the computer in the observation room where the technician was safely working the spaceship-like machinery. I held still for fifteen minutes, but I didn't have to worry about my breathing because the freaky computer even accounted for those variations. The technology boggled my mind every time.

Each time, I heard the funny language of the radiation emitter spinning into its precise position charted by the computer program. And each time, while it whirred and whined, I marveled about this technology and felt enormous gratitude for the geniuses who invented it. I also felt sad for all the men who in previous times never had this advantage. This disease now being nuked into oblivion had killed millions of my brothers and broken the hearts of millions of their loved ones. The enormity of it often made me weep as I lay there getting saved.

"Thank You, God, for this lifesaving high-tech equipment, for the doctors who have learned how to use it, and for the technicians who deliver the radiation. And thank You for my courage to take this on and stay with it in the face of uncertainty."

My testosterone plummeted and would stay down for five or six months. The side effects soared: I lost sexual function, physical stamina, and body hair; hot flashes and weight gain added to my general discomfort; and my breasts became tender and enlarged. My endocrine system was turned upside down, and so was my lifestyle.

In mid-December, two weeks after finishing the external radiation, I stayed overnight in the hospital for the radioactive seed implants, which went directly into my prostate. A spinal anesthetic made the procedure itself painless. Although I didn't much like lying on my back postoperatively for several hours, I was willing to do it because that prevented a spinal headache. Besides, I was distracted for the first hour in the recovery room by the

193

nurse asking my advice about what to do about her husband's moodiness and irritability.

All in all, the whole deal initially seemed like a piece of cake, especially with Susan's constant ministrations. It wasn't until the anesthesia wore off that the catheter became awkward. I took it like a trooper until early the following morning when I was liberated by its removal, dependent on resumption of spontaneous urine production. I was glad to leave. Off we drove to the doctor's clinic for post-op X-rays and then home. It was on the way home from the hospital that I promised to record this experience from start to finish.

I passed blood (as predicted) on the first day. I hit the gym on day two, and every day thereafter. Full-time office hours resumed after my resting at home over the weekend.

Once in place, the radioactive seeds were designed to deliver a precise dose of radiation to exact spots over three or four months. As they were saving my life, however, they extracted the price of raging side effects, which became the butt of jokes between Susan and me and the bane of our lifestyle. But again, "They beat the box."

But is all this treatment really saving me, or is it just adding well-meant insults to injury? Is this a schtick that I'm putting myself through, or will it be worth it?

Absent a crystal ball, I had no viable choice but to do all that I could do and hope for the best—and not hold my breath in the meantime. Both Susan and I had to ignore the scythe hanging up there, hoping that all the medical efforts and my unending praying, meditating, and introspecting would pay off. That posture required daily reinforcement in a way that was not obsessive and did not take the foreground. I wanted to live life fully, whatever I had left of it.

Now make life work as best you can, my man. And don't be haunted by uncertainty. That's life. Just look around. Everybody's showing up with hurts and fears inside. The result won't be in until you arrive at the box. For as long as you have, go for it.

195

Chapter 15
Six-Month Follow-Up

So far, so good. First obstacle cleared, but a lot of marathon left, with many pit stops. Plenty of laughs, too.

After several weeks, the implanted radiation seeds began to slowly dissipate so that by the end of four months they were lifeless and inactive. Then they just sit there forever and amuse radiologists who happen upon them when looking for other things. That's the nuclear physics part.

But the fun started for me in December, the first week that the seeds were doing their job (as I've said, the game definitely was on). Short-term steroids in the first few days helped a bit with the prostate inflammation and related obstruction symptoms, but the real story over the ensuing eighteen months was that my symptoms exploded and were more extreme than in most cases. No matter, because the main point here was my response to their challenge, not

197

their severity, not to mention that I was alive and might remain so—even early on, I had the sense that I'd made it, or at least I had cultivated an attitude that believed it. So I just took care of business.

At the far end of the distribution curve of severity, my angry prostate began to give me grief day and night—especially night. I peed hot burning tacks every thirty to forty-five minutes, day and night, for what turned out to be at least eighteen months. Then it dropped to every hour or hour and a half or so for another six months. I became accustomed to carrying a urinal in the car and keeping a supply of Kotex handy. Since my wife did not sleep like a rock, I had relocated to the guest bedroom. Fifteen bathroom trips a night was not uncommon. Yes, the game was on big time.

The other possible side effects of my combination of treatments were many, And I experienced most of them. Some of the more taxing included fatigue, reduced stamina, weight gain, painful breast enlargement, loss of libido and sexual function, hot flashes, insomnia, and all the urinary symptoms in spades. It was a daunting list, at least in my case. Thankfully, though, I did not become depressed or slowed in my thinking. I was tired but not knocked down, not by a long shot. I kept up my morning workouts at the gym, and most of my professional and personal life carried on. But when the urinary symptoms hit, they posed more of a challenge than I'd anticipated. My measure was taken every day and every night, 24/7, but that was the deal. As long as I could be as effective as ever in patient care, I was on; in fact, I had never been more empathic. And—no small thing—I was alive.

There were some significant sacrifices, though none as dire as losing my sight or my ability to walk or speak or, by the way, dying.

When I reminded myself of that perspective and when I thought of the alternative, I went through nothing. But I had to put a moratorium on anything that required my uninterrupted attention for more than thirty minutes. My appointment schedule allowed that without a problem, but my love life? My wife and I both had to settle for nothing more than cuddling affection.

There were places where I had to look for help. I could see patients, but inevitably my staff had to help me with scheduling patients around my treatments and seeing to it that I wasn't bothered with minutiae that, when healthy, I had handled without even thinking about it. If you have good people around you, this can usually be done almost seamlessly. Luckily I have and it did.

The same was true for our friends. It's practically a cliché to say that when disaster strikes, real friends present themselves while the rest send a card or make one quick phone call. Cliché or not, the statement seemed true. One lifeline was the telephone—no wonder one telephone company's advertisement used to say "Reach out and touch someone." I'm sure other cancer patients heard those words and know how true they are.

As the side effects escalated, I did my best to make sure I talked to our kids and our friends. Sometimes I had a specific reason to call, but if none came to mind and I just needed to talk, I called. The phone was also important to Susan. After all, she was often stuck there with me and had her own need to hear fresh voices. She did share with me some aspects of her side of the picture, but I'm sure she lowballed it out of trying to mitigate my concern about being a boring, stay-at-home evening "veg" who was running back and forth to the bathroom. But she had her friends and family with whom I knew she was venting.

For example, the imposition of my particular degree of

symptoms forced us to curtail some of our favorite activities. They were small prices to pay for my life, but no one had forewarned me. Unless I wanted to disturb everyone around me every twenty or thirty minutes, two-hour performances were out. This applied to movies, concerts, and sports events.

And forget fishing. It would be unimaginable to try leaning out over the transom of a boat, doing the prostate dance, wiggling, pulling, straining, and cursing in plain view of your fishing buddies as nearly nothing comes out. Do that for five minutes? Every twenty or thirty minutes? And then the barbs and jokes to dispel the tension? No thanks.

To alleviate being bored or irritated at the losses of some outlets, I held onto which ever ones I could. Writing was one; two others were meditation and workouts, which had always been part of my schedule. Even though interruptions were necessary for bathroom breaks, they didn't keep me from my (somewhat altered) routine. These activities were important for stress reduction.

Also, although we had to stop going out, that didn't mean we couldn't have friends over, and we went to their homes as well. Once again, our friends were great about this. They knew the limitations I was under and didn't mind if I had to excuse myself several times in the course of an evening. Even at that, those evenings were shorter than they would have been under normal circumstances.

I've always been teased for going to bed early, and in the past fifteen years or so, I haven't liked staying out past 10:00 or 10:30 P.M. even on weekends. I would always rise at 5:30 to work out. But these days, the treatments and required regimens often left me tired by day's end, sometimes to the point of exhaustion. Most evenings, I would be in bed asleep by 8:30 P.M., leaving Susan alone.

As I've heard about others' experiences, it strikes me that the post-treatment discomfort and life interferences are not usually in the range I encountered. But I repeatedly remind myself that the name of the game on my cancer journey is to face the Great Mystery over and over and to persevere in rebounding. The severity of my own particulars only emphasizes the challenge and my chance to prove myself.

Susan's tolerance and goodwill were tested by many things, including my need for a nearby bathroom. As I've said, going out to parties, restaurants, or events meant an "Excuse me" every few minutes and the rush to make the bathroom in time. And then, if the john was occupied, painful urgency could turn into a very difficult situation, quickly changing our night out into an exasperating, embarrassing, and short-lived exercise. For months, our home, which had always been our sanctuary, was far more of a center of life than it ever had been before. While we'd always enjoyed being at home, nothing could hide the stifling feeling of not going wherever we wanted. It wasn't much fun. But hey…

They say that faith is forged in the fire. It's true. My faith in love, God, and self must focus on how I play the game, not on the scoreboard. There is no scoreboard. This isn't a game of points, runs, or baskets, and I'm not waiting for a buzzer. I need to muster the internal stuff—courage and honor—and persevere. Of course I hope to win, to stay alive.

How many hundreds of times was I to remind myself of this in the wee hours of the morning as I winced at the night's tenth urinary crisis?

Fighting the good fight is its own reward, my man. Do it right and never let up. The winning is in the process, Bob. You win, even if you lose.

With that attitude, winning came with each moment. My foresight extended to the next PSA test and little further. I didn't excessively grieve over the health I'd enjoyed in the recent past; instead, I dealt with the issues at hand. I was growing up.

Staying power required "juice"—physical, emotional, and spiritual. As the radiation and drugs took their toll, my physical energy and stamina became more and more depleted, especially at the end of the day. Yet somehow my clinical work remained constant, as did my exercise and meditation. The most important sustaining "juice" came from love and faith as well as regular cackles, snickers, guffaws, or whatever else I could come up with.

Nothing broke tension or reset my perspective like a well-placed jest. I didn't use laughter to deflect or deny sadness or anger, but I appreciated wit and a sense of irony. Funny moments dispelled the tendency to feel sad, thereby helping me to avoid feeling sorry for myself. In effect, well-placed humor was a protection against victimhood. For my family and me, poking fun has been more than mere style; it has always been a natural way to stay honest. Our friends and my staff also understood humor's usefulness in diffusing tension and avoiding denial.

Susan and I had a running joke that it would be early summer, after the testosterone dive started to let up, before I awoke from the dead, which was the four- to six-month predicted duration for Lupron shutdown. Little did we know at the time that the prostate had other ideas. We decided the extra pounds must have meant that the castrating treatment had gone a step further—making me pregnant. The breast enlargement fell right into the Seinfeld episode of the "bro," a brassiere for men.

******

Sometimes the funniest moments were the most painful, such as when my angry prostate would terrorize me while commuting. I learned to use my own GPS to measure "pee intervals." My pee mileage was five miles on the highway, two miles in traffic. More than any fill-up, that defined my coming and going.

Many evenings when returning home from the office, I would cut it close, knowing that I couldn't afford a traffic snarl. Oftentimes the traffic slowed but didn't halt, but slowing down was alarming enough. Teetering on the very brink of meltdown, I would barely make it to the bushes in front of the house, where I would reduce our innocent shrubs from tropical décor to emergency urinals.

One evening, my commuter's urinary crisis was nearing its peak as I made the final turn toward the island of Siesta Key. At that moment I saw the drawbridge ahead start to rise.

Shit!

I took a sharp left turn onto a side street. Plastic urinal in hand, I frantically searched for the first available deserted section of street. I'd already unfastened my seat belt, sending the alert into its "screech" phase, and the prostate tyrant threatened to explode any second. At each side street I began to anticipate relief—I just needed a minute to sneak out the plastic urinal right then and there behind the wheel. Then came a jogger...

Shit!...Shit!!

On another night, it was someone walking a dog. I found myself wishing I was the pooch who could pee in public without drawing scrutiny. These desperate forays into side streets didn't always end in victory. More than once I met defeat, first with curses but then with peals of laughter. On several evenings, as I walked into the house soaked and chagrined, Susan roared.

She guffawed at a lot of things: my proud announcements that I had a "twenty-five pee day" or nights that I could claim a "fifteener." Sometimes I topped that. The television commercial about "Gotta go, gotta go" took on a depth and relevance we'd never dreamed it could have—and hoped it would never have again. It became our chant as I took on the motto: "Urinals are my life." I jokingly considered starting my own stand-up comedy act. The material was there, but my sets would have to be on the short side.

To make it through all of the side effects and the ongoing fear of the Reaper lurking in the background, I relied on active spiritual practice. My morale had to remain solid in order to get through each day at my best. I'd never faced the imminence of my own death before; no doubt such urgency had propelled my rapid growth from a child-like perspective to adulthood. In many ways I was ready, given my internal changes over the years. As I thought about it, the timing was right for the wake-up call. I had grown a lot and just needed the kick in the ass from cancer to push me up into the next level of maturity.

In certain ways, I faced a choice between faith and failure: fight or quit. Since faith had played an increasingly positive role in my development for the past twenty years, I was primed for the cancer call. I was generally optimistic and grounded. It was as if the leftover adolescent habits and naiveté were ripe for the plucking.

I was learning quickly the difference between immature and mature prayer. No matter how hard I prayed or how positively I held intention, it was obvious that I had no control over outcomes. It didn't matter how good a guy I was or what professional standing I'd earned; the good boy's prayer wasn't going to get me a cure—I kept on peeing hot tacks. And even regarding my attitude, it was obvious that God wouldn't do much for me unless I was willing to do things for myself. For instance, in the face of uncertainty, I had to take whatever came and make the best of it. The unacceptable option was to fold, a maxim I'd preached to my patients for years.

Now can I practice my own teachings? Can I focus on my Serenity Prayer and concentrate on each of those things that can be done? Am I going to show up every day?

Those questions plagued me. In meditative prayer, I found positive answers or at least accommodation. After six decades plus, I was still learning and changing. Though my prayers were no longer those of the star, the good little boy, I still believed that good must rule in this world, even if it wasn't obvious to me at the moment, especially at 3:00 A.M. clutching the side of the bathroom sink and preparing myself for the imminent searing shot. Of course newspapers and TV news don't help much with a positive view of humankind, and much of history doesn't either, so I made sure that I saw a balanced big picture in order to hold my positive sense about life and about my particular struggle with the mystery. My meditation reminded me of life's wondrous beauty and infinite intelligence.

Sometimes that was easier said than done. At exasperating times I had the urge to "throw the baby out with the bathwater," as the cliché goes. But I kept in mind the Rule of Holes: There's trouble enough already. I prayed for courage and strength, stayed with the mystery, and accepted my impotence. In accepting it, I also realized that I did have control of some things: my level of play, my preparedness for any outcome, and my determination not to bang my head against a wall. As a friend once told me, "You can't choose the cards you're dealt, including whether or not you deserve them, but you can decide how to play your hand."

Isn't that how life itself works? Nothing ventured, nothing gained. Music, plays, movies, books, and artwork of all kinds send that message over and over, but there's nothing like your own trial by fire. How can truth be discovered without getting burned?

Show up, and God and love will do the rest.

It's never an easy lesson, but it was particularly hard for the star.

******

When faith reaches maturity, our prayers no longer assume that God will take care of everything. I would pray something like this:

I come to Your loving and kind embrace to ask for support and loving acceptance. I am never alone, for You are always there. I ask You to enhance my appreciation of life's beauty as I celebrate the chance to be fully alive. I resonate with Your healing, loving energy, which is always available in infinite supply. I am one with my brothers and sisters in acceptance and wonder at who they are, each a unique being in humanity and spirit. I accept the ugly as part of life's full palette. It helps me to see the beauty more clearly.

Help me to have the courage to dare to be fully alive. Help me to be fully present each day at my personal best. As I do the best that I can, be with me through the light and the dark. I draw on Your infinite strength and wisdom to make my choices, and I count on Your loving support to help me keep my faith, hold my purpose, and stay open in heart and spirit. And I'll do my best to keep enough humility to be able to take myself with a grain of salt, even when I'm most fervent and earnest. I'll try to stop banging my head against the wall and struggling to get control over events. And last but not least, I'll search for every healing grin and laugh I can find. Amen.

For me, all of those concepts had come into play. I was losing physical strength daily; I needed more rest than I once had; I was gaining weight, bloating, and losing my libido; and I had to change shirts in the evenings because of the sweat from my hot flashes. That's when Susan would make a crack that a man with prostate cancer can finally know what every woman goes through without a fuss. "Welcome to my world," she teased. I couldn't help but laugh in my exasperation.

No description really prepared me. I'd been warned about every detail, but I'd been certain that those details really didn't apply to me. I was the guy who would beat the symptoms, the one who would dodge every side effect. The side effects would be few and they would be fairly minimal, or maybe they'd hardly be there at all. I was to be the star patient, the good boy whom God looked after, so I would be spared.

Gag.

In retrospect, I was embarrassed to have been so childish. It turned out that my so-called passage on the beach was just a beginning because naturally I hadn't grown up in an hour. Indeed, such a child-like idea would, in and of itself, be telling. There I was, months later, still with the post-treatment challenges, all day and all night.

It has been humbling to recall that I'd assumed that I would be mature and would have the kind of expectations of God and say the type of prayer any adult would offer: the Serenity Prayer. While I used to advise others to consider it, I found that deep down I was really like a third grader. All I needed was a cancerous prostate to wake me up—and it did, every twenty minutes, day and night.

As the mini-crises of making it to the bathroom took

over every hour of my life, each small situation gave me the opportunity to choose: I could reaffirm my positive perspective amidst the laughing and the cursing, or I could get angry and fed up, throwing it all out as bullshit and psychobabble. I made sure that I did the former.

Humor came hardest at three in the morning, during my umpteenth struggle to bring a precious ounce from the prostate fires. But even then, I sometimes burst out laughing. It was the only thing to do.

******

Despite the cancer, my practice went well—in some ways better than ever. My empathy was deepening as I felt more and more a part of the universal struggle with life's fragility. Thankfully, I was able to structure patients around the little dictator, and usually my appointment schedule fit with the timing of his demands.

Evenings weren't so easy. For Susan and me, not being able to go out was frustrating enough, but we couldn't even have evening walks together. Walking stimulates the bladder, and a hundred yards from the front door I had to turn around. That wasn't relaxing. Another thing was the hot tub, which we used to use daily because those massaging currents would relax us from the day's action. But alas, no hot tub because it heats up the prostate tyrant, so for a year it was good-bye to the hot tub. Shopping with Susan for things for the house dropped off my immediate to-do list. We often had enjoyed an afternoon of looking for antiques, but that was not happening. Tennis and biking were also out.

Thankfully, Susan is her own woman and kept her own activities going. I couldn't travel to see either of my newborn grandsons or my other three grandchildren. Of course, the grown children understood, but I feared that I was fading from the younger ones' memories. Phone calls can't quite replace physical presence.

But after all was weighed on the balance scale, these accommodations were nothing compared to the alternative—talk about keeping perspective and counting blessings. With humor and love, life did indeed go forward.

Chapter 16

New Year's Day 2005

Looking decent. Another couple of laboratory hurdles are cleared. Small lifestyle challenges every day.

At one year post-treatment, the daily exasperations and laughs had become my life. Susan was right there in the trenches with me, and I was putting up a pretty good fight. I hadn't missed a day at the office, nor had I missed a workout. My body went right on with its endocrine changes, so I put on weight, grew tender breasts, and lost my libido and related functions. No one but Susan knew. But I remained sharp and lively enough to put in a full day at my practice, and my enhanced empathy had improved my doctoring. My staff was upbeat and positive, telling me that my level of function hadn't fallen off. Of course one of the funny ones—taking a cue from me—had to add, "That is, for a dying man."

******

One day I sat on the deck early in the morning, basking in the warm sun. The sky was a cloudless light blue, the lagoon glistened, and a cormorant dived for his meal. I lapsed into recent memories about my two trips to the doctors for follow-up verdicts: one at six months and the most recent at twelve months. Nothing in my life compared to either of them; never had I gone to get an answer as important. Even at that, neither result was necessarily final or determinative, so even two years was too soon to let out my breath.

In retrospect, the only events that came close in terms of a crisis were going to court twenty-four years previously to set divorce parameters and attending an IRS hearing for the humiliating and infuriating determination of an uncalled-for Chapter 13 just because my pockets were deeper than the real culprit's. Both called for seeing the big picture, staying positive, and making sure to avoid lapsing into cynicism.

But in the past two years, my life had been on the line, with much higher stakes. And I was reminded every day, all day, by the relentless side effects of treatment, which were in full swing at both six months and twelve months post-treatment. But I was making it; I hadn't taken so much as a knee.

******

The six-month reality check came upon me. I was to go in for the blood tests and color flow Doppler and get the answer about my life or death, at least the probabilities at that point in time.

Our evening at home before the next day's

212

pronouncement was uneventful for Susan and me, except for the unspoken apprehension in both of us. I had, of course, told her of the upcoming tests, and her response was her usual positive one: "You'll be OK. And if not, we'll think about it then. For now, just get a good night's sleep, sweetheart." She gave me a big reassuring hug, and I went off to bed a bit earlier than usual.

The next office day was straightforward because I had successfully put the issue on the back burner. On only a couple of occasions that day did a patient talk about awaiting a lab result, one of which had been no less than a determinative breast cancer biopsy. I couldn't help shuddering a bit at the thought of her walking into an office and getting an answer like I was about to. But as so often had been the case, her courage set an example for me.

My appointment was for 4:30, the last of my doctor's day. I liked to schedule it that way in case he was running late because at least I wouldn't have to worry about my patients waiting for me in my office. I couldn't stand to keep them waiting; this way, the issue was moot. It was a half hour away, with a ten-minute drive to get there...

Plenty of time, my friend.

As I bid the last patient a good day, I began to feel a bit woozy. My legs wobbled and my heart rate quickened so that I could feel it fluttering in my neck and chest. I sat down in my office chair for a mini-meditation, just enough to set my intention and my attitude and to ratchet up my courage. That done, I stood up on firm feet, my chest stuck out, and my head erect. Out I went to the car and drove off to my verdict.

Other moments, including two court experiences, surgery for skin cancer, my first day at MGH, and even marriage and childbirth, paled in comparison. This moment was the one in which I would learn whether I would be alive only a bit longer or a lot longer. My research had already revealed that this early follow-up would not be a definitive test for the long term, but it would tell me whether the atom bomb appeared to have done its demolition work, at least for this stage, or had missed its target.

"So far, so good," my doctor announced from his position at my feet as he stared at the color flow Doppler video image. I was hiked up in the stirrups like a woman getting a pelvic exam. What must have been an entire X-ray machine was inserted in my rectum—actually, it was merely a high-tech camera, a modern marvel designed to visualize blood vessels, the life supply of cancer. No cancer tissue would escape detection. A monitor was positioned near my head so that I could watch while listening to his ongoing commentary.

He went on to tell me that the gland had shrunk to so many grams and that the dark areas were where the cancer had been. He showed me pretreatment images to compare. Yes, indeed, now there was black where there used to be color. "Whew," I exhaled audibly. He got my drift and said that this was a good study for this stage, six months post-treatment.

"We're right on track," he told me. Then he picked up my chart. "Your labs look good. Your PSA is undetectable, which is nice to see."

That's putting it mildly.

"So it's too early to call this a cure, but everything looks real good. I'll see you back in six more months for your one-year follow-up. If that's as good as this, we'll be even more pleased."

I must admit that a small naïve part of my positive self was a bit let down. I knew better, but I wanted the battle to be over. Of course it wasn't—and wouldn't be, even in a year. But with every six months of good results, the chances of relapse or persistence became more and more remote. His voluminous clinical research data showed negligible risk at three or more years.

So in the parking lot I called Susan with the news.

"Honey, it's not bad, and it's not wonderful."

"OK, how about in English?"

"What I mean is, as of today, there's no sign of cancer. And in another six months, or especially a year or two, we'll really know. So for now, it's good."

"That's great. We'll take one step at a time. What was it you always said about not knowing the score until you played the game? Come on home to me."

******

Moving into the one-year follow-up, the story was much the same. My endocrine symptoms were on the wane, so no more night sweats or hot flashes. My breasts had returned to normal, but my libido had not—still just cuddling and affection. But the inflammation roared along, keeping me constantly vigilant for men's rooms. Our lives were still structured around pee intervals, but our spirits were good and we kept laughing whenever we could find a twist or a sick joke.

But I approached the one-year Doppler exam and blood work results with a different kind of apprehension compared to that of the six-month follow-up. The longer-term evaluation was about the endurance of the results.

Has it returned? Is my PSA still undetectable? Has our struggle been in vain against a relentless killer?

This time I was looking for still being in the ball game and winning by a bigger margin.

"This looks great," exclaimed my doctor from down

there around my feet as I lay supine, spread-eagle, on the table. Yes indeed, there it was on the monitor, a black area where there used to be cancer.

Yes!! I pumped my fist jubilantly. I'm still in this one!

He went on to explain that indeed I was and that my PSA was still undetectable, a favorable sign because some men have a bit of a rise at this point, even though they go on to do well. In fact, all I needed at that point were labs in six months and a Doppler study plus labs in a year. Light at the tunnel's end came into view.

******

Whew. Have I made it? I'm looking good so far. It's been well over a year, and the labs are good. I'm still peeing hot tacks, but that's the deal, I'm told. The Reaper is only a passing thought now. Screw him and his scythe.

Chapter 17

Blood on the Sheets

Just when my hopes started to rise...Ba da bing! What the hell is this?

I threw back the covers to rise and take on another day at the office. I felt fairly refreshed because my urinary symptoms were lessening after eighteen months. Those days, sleep interruptions were down to six to eight or so at night, compared to twice that amount a year prior. I had just thrown my legs over the side of the bed, preparing to step onto the floor when I saw them—brilliant spots of red, a few dime-sized circular spots with many smaller spots nearby. As best as I can figure, all were at the level of my waist as I lay in the bed, on the bottom sheet and top sheet as well.

Oh, shit. This wasn't in the list of expected side effects.

Before panicking about the spread of cancer to the bladder, I reverted to basic medical thinking. If this were in the bladder, the urine would be mixed with blood. If it were from the prostate, pure red blood could be expressed from the penile opening without first mixing with urine upstream. It would have been the first liquid out. Thanks to all the saints, the latter was the case. I could express a drop of pure red blood; nonetheless, this needed investigating. Only then did my breathing slow and my panic lessen...a bit.

My God, will this never end? How long am I to live with this sword hanging over my head? Come on, God, what are You up to?

Sure enough, my radiation oncologist wanted a urology consult. In the meantime, he sent a special urine specimen to the cytology lab to look for cancer cells. I also got an intravenous pyelogram (IVP), in which dye is injected into a forearm vein and time is allowed for the kidney to filter it out into the drainage system, thereby lighting up the X-rays of the entire urinary tract from the kidneys down to the bladder. And all that time, I (like everyone else undergoing medical tests) had to go on with life as normal.

Those test results were within normal limits: no cancer mass in the bladder, no backup distension, no pressure buildup in the system. Those were good. I had waited for those results with not a little private pacing and hand-wringing. And what the hell, I threw in some little boy prayers for good results and some mature prayers for courage.

By the time I saw the urologist, I was at least reassured that the urine cytology had shown no cancer cells and that the IVP was okay. But I dreaded the possibility of having to undergo a cystogram, which would involve yet another intrusive procedure of shoving a pipe through my penis up into my bladder, inserting a camera through it, having a look around, and taking biopsies of anything suspicious.

Seriously, it wouldn't be all that traumatic, but I was just fed up with mechanical objects being thrust into my rectum and penis. Frankly, we men have known little of the intrusive exams and instrumentation procedures that women have routinely gone through for years. When he told me that the history, urine analysis, and IVP were enough, I was—to say the least—relieved. For now, I had a reprieve, but I would need yearly urine tests for cytology, just to make sure that the cancer hadn't spread.

Swell.

******

"Excuse me, sir, the seat belt sign is still on. The pilot has not indicated that passengers may get up and walk about the cabin."

"Miss, I'm not trying to be defiant. It's just that I have no choice but to make that lavatory in about three seconds. I'll explain later," I blurted on my way lurching up the aisle to the tiny place labeled lavatory. My prostate, the great equalizer, cared nothing for accommodations or conditions; it just demanded attention. Remember—gardens, napkins, diapers, and shrubs had all served in the past two years. And after all that, there I was, occasionally bleeding, and I was still frantically scrambling for the plane's men's room. The absurdity of the scene nearly sent me into guffaws crouched right there in front of the head in the two-by-two closet called a lavatory into which I had crammed myself. Air motion jostled me up and down, making accurate aim more difficult than usual, given the need to jump in place and manipulate my poor beleaguered organ.

You gotta be kidding me.

I just didn't want to run the gauntlet back down the aisle with my pants wet and my face red. The flight

219

attendant never asked for any further explanation, so my plight must have been self-explanatory.

What sit-com material.

Scenes like that in the second year reflected our being adventuresome enough to travel to Rhode Island, where we took refuge in our dear little stone cottage. We also ventured out in the car for trips of an hour or two, as long as I had scoped out the men's rooms along the route, but just in case, I had my trusty urinal in the car. God forbid I had to use it, though, because Susan would shriek with laughter and pull some prank or another, threatening to embarrass me. Then I would be laughing so hard I couldn't concentrate enough on the prostate dance, the little jig I had to perform in place just to get something started.

After about three or four weeks of intermittent bleeding, the inflammation slowed and the red spots stopped. Then I lived with trying to decide whether it was over or just an intermission. Would I resume hemorrhaging at any time? Would I spot from time to time? How long would I have to check my underwear and sheets? Forever? It turned out that I did spot several weeks later, but that was pretty much it. For more than a year, I continued checking the sheets and my underwear for the dreaded red signal.

******

The rest of the second year settled down to minor symptoms and few intrusions into our lifestyle. We resumed our walks, tennis, movie and theater nights, and travel. My nightly pees were reduced to three or four per night, few enough for us to get a decent night's sleep together

After the first year or so, no one mentioned the cancer or inquired about my status, except dear friends from out of the area whom we saw only periodically; they, of course, wanted to catch up. I showed no distress or symptoms of illness, so it was as if nothing had happened. Meanwhile, I took nothing for granted; I had to stay on top of my game, even as the score seemed to gradually improve. I knew that I couldn't take much of a breath until the three-year checkup, and even then it was not a forever guarantee. But what was?

Before the third-year checkup, some lab tests were required at two and a half years. My PSA continued to be undetectable, as did the urine cytology for cancer cells. Certainly I was relieved each time my tests were normal, but every time I called for results, my heart was in my throat.

With cancer, it ain't over 'til it's over.

The real question, though, was at what point would the probability of recurrence bottom out to resemble that of just living this life? Meanwhile, I tried to live my life without much thought about danger. Our lifestyle normalized, or at least we could come and go as we pleased. I did a local TV show on bouncing back from cancer, so it was no longer a secret. Some patients had watched it and expressed their surprise, since I hadn't seemed ill. When dealing with a cancer victim, I occasionally offered at least the fact that I was having post-cancer treatment and apparently surviving. I didn't go into details in the clinical context because, after all, their needs were the focus, not mine. But from their reactions to even a brief sharing of the fact of our common experience, I could tell that they were grateful for my brief candor.

So compared to the first two years of active reminders and compromises, the third year was more like a reprieve. Was it denial? Was it positive thinking and strong faith? I preferred to believe the latter. But even though life was taking on an ordinary feel, there still lurked the reality of the three-year prostate study that was to mark the point in the risk curve that would be telling. If cancer were to recur, it would most likely happen by then. If I were in the clear, I should get a pretty good prognosis at that point. No guarantees about this or anything else, but it would suggest whether I was at least on my way to freedom for a while.

******

Now I'm about to find out.

Part 4

The Moment of Truth

Chapter 18

The Moment of Truth

THE trial. Either the Grim Reaper wins, or I win and he is on his way out. Decision: I win!

T he day had finally arrived. I would get my verdict of life or death—well, maybe not that dramatic, but damned close. For instance, if there were a recurrence, I was dead, sooner rather than later, but if not, maybe I'd have an ordinary life span unrelated to the cancer. Never had I faced such a pronouncement. Even the first six-month workup paled in comparison. My trying to live a productive life in the face of pain and limitations had been part of a waiting game.

I've been holding my breath for three years while trying to live fully every day. So has Susan. Now we'll get our answer.

I'd visited the children and grandchildren and celebrated Christmases, birthdays, and other family events as if I were fine. Later, family members confessed that early on they could see how strained and wan I'd get, especially after a lot of activity. But no one let on back then. I'd attended many hundreds of patients with even greater skill. None of them had said anything until I went public with a TV show and several articles on surviving cancer; then a few volunteered that I'd seemed a bit tired in the first year or so.

I even saw beauty where I hadn't before, and I surely didn't sweat the small stuff. I tried to shed the pounds I'd gained but had no success, despite continued workouts. Susan and I were closer than ever because we had shared one of life's terrors. I was even writing on a regular basis after a workday and on weekends since my energy had resumed its characteristic inexhaustibility.

But the Grim Reaper's shadow always hovered in the back of my mind, so to speak, and it did in the back of Susan's as well. I was both aware of my mortality and aware of the need to make every moment count. To say the least, much of the learning from these three years was spiritual: facing the unanswerable, seeing the apparent injustice, and coming up more joyous, more loving. The enhanced awareness of risk had led to more openness, not retreat.

All of that said, for three years I was still scared. But the day arrived to face the music.

******

I checked the sheets like always. Nope, no blood. Every day since that trauma a year and a half ago, I still checked the sheets. I rolled out of bed, stretched, and, like always, dressed for my morning workout. Also, even three years later, I always checked the force, initiation, and stopping of

226

the urine stream.

No problem.

But today I had butterflies and a queasy stomach and was tired, since I hadn't slept well. Thankfully, I couldn't recall the details of some weird dreams, but there was something about drowning in the ocean or not making it to the boat.

Nice way to start out this day of all days.

But as always, I gathered myself and went through the day without showing any sign of what I was feeling as I approached the 4:00 P.M. judgment hour at my doctor's office. Susan had given me a big hug and reassurances the night before. She insisted on the obvious, which was that I call her as soon as I heard the word. I'd tucked away my apprehension for my own survival. I didn't want emotional flooding to intrude into my work with patients or my interactions with staff. Also, I'd resolved not to obsess.

At 3:30 P.M. the time had arrived to go, so I said my cheery good-byes to my staff and went out to my car. Once I was strapped in, the doors to my compartmentalized feelings began to open. One by one they emerged: fear, apprehension, sorrow, anger, impotence, bewilderment, and more. I was clearly at the mercy of whatever was in store for me in thirty minutes. My first task was to drive there safely, so I used that to focus; the rest was held at bay. I made it safely to the doctor's parking lot.

Then my breathing revved up, and so did my heart rate. I gripped the wheel tightly in order to feel a sensation that I could will and focus on as a way into some calm. A few long deep breaths and I was back in charge, at least of some of my functions. So I got out of the car on wobbly legs— walking over to the office door was like stepping on a sponge. By the time I grasped the handle to swing open the door, I was out of breath.

227

This door weighs a thousand pounds. I'm about to enter some chamber of either mercy or torture. I'll soon know.

The experience was much worse than the day I came home to Susan after the beach walk. Entering the house that day was heavy, but at least I was about to encounter one sure thing: loving resolve. Besides, at that point the journey was just getting underway, with all of the excitement and terror of taking on the unknown. And this moment was more terrifying than any of my follow-up exams over the past three years. Now I was going to get my answer after three years of sustained effort—my verdict.

The ponderous door swung open despite my passing fantasy that maybe it would be stuck or that the office had closed early. A cheerful member of the office staff greeted me at the front desk, much as she would if she were working at a flower shop.

"Hi, I'm Doctor Mignone. I have an appointment at 4:30 with the doctor to see if I'm going to live or die."

"Hi, I'm Doctor Mignone, here for my 4:30 appointment."

I sat and waited ten interminable minutes before being called into the inner sanctum. The formally appointed waiting room was funeral parlor–like that day.

I was back in the pelvic exam position amidst lighthearted banter from the tech about the Bucs and Red Sox. In came the man who would pronounce me dead or alive, and he too was business as usual. I felt weightless, as if floating in a space capsule. This time I couldn't bear to watch the monitor as he and the tech talked in sotto voce with one another.

Are they finding cancer? Such low tones must be ominous. If the picture were so good, they'd be exclaiming already. Steady, Bob...

Of course I realized that they were carefully evaluating

the images and discussing findings just as they should.
*But why can't they do so without my hearing their
ambiguous exchange? They're taking hours. Damn this
suspense.*

My heart rate began to pick up. So did my breathing.
What the hell is it?

"This is as good as it gets," the doctor announced with
obvious pleasure. "Your PSA is still undetectable, your
symptoms are negligible, and this study continues to show
no cancer after three years. I hate to say the word 'cure,'
but this is as close as it can be."

Well, I could have jumped up and hugged him right
then and there. Instead, I fought back tears of relief and
said, "Thank you! Thank you for saving my life!" It was all
I could do to suppress sobs. He modestly sidestepped my
unabashed gratitude by crediting the modern equipment
and my steadfast participation, to which I repeated, "Yes,
yes, but thank you for saving my life."

I strolled out of his office and through the waiting area,
which seemed dressed up like a resort hotel lobby, walking
six inches off the ground and feeling light as a feather. I
floated over to my awaiting Beemer chariot silhouetted
against a setting sun, and it was an especially beautiful
piece of sculpture—in fact, everything around me was
bigger, richer, more alive, and more vibrant than ever
before. I entered the car, picked up my cell phone, and
called Susan.

"Beemer to Susan. Beemer to Susan. The eagle has
landed. I'm going to live. I'm going to live! All three years
of troubles were worth it. I'm going to make it, baby!"

"That's just wonderful, sweetheart! I'm so happy for
both of us. Get home here quick. I knew this would be OK,
so I bought a bottle of champagne and some sushi. We'll
sip and munch in the hot tub."

"I'm on my way, darling. I should be there in no time. And, my dear wife, I can never thank you enough for everything."

"Of course you can, darling. We'll talk. By the way, your old idea about a commemorative diamond sounds interesting, yes? As an investment, I mean…"

I threw back my head and for the first time in three years had a real laugh that had no element of gallows humor.

******

Yes! You gottaluvit!!

Chapter 19

Our Dear Little Stone Cottage

So don't think it's over. It ain't ever over. Just the specifics change. The marathon's finish line is the box.

Our stone cottage in coastal Rhode Island has been our continuing connection with our cultural backgrounds, kids, and grandchildren. Built in 1911, it has remained a quintessential piece of New England, constructed from stones gathered from clearing the fields used to farm or breed dairy cows. Rhode Island is especially known for its stone walls made from the bounty of generous glaciers. It has been our little getaway, our base from which to visit our friends and family. When we bought it, there were only two bedrooms, a kitchen, and a large living room with a woodstove. A Rube Goldberg add-on porch served us at the rear, facing toward the backyard and a meadow beyond.

The adorable stone structure sat in the lee of hillside

woods. In the front, a narrow lane wound up the hill on which we were set; just over the wooded hill and down the other side was the water, Narragansett Bay, named the Sakonnet River at that point in Tiverton. For years our small sheltered cove has been a haven for boats at mooring. A small beach has offered opportunities for bathing in private, throwing pebbles, launching our little boat, or just plain sitting back and taking in nature. Looking to the south was nature conservancy land, and across the wide expanse of water were dots of homes on the Portsmouth side.

We had given this special place new life with an architect and a local builder experienced in antique houses. It was doubled in size, though it retains the same look and feel of an old New England cottage. Although we had to take a hiatus of more than a year and a half during its construction work, recently we were again able to sit on the porch and reflect on life and nonsense.

******

One early morning I was alone on our new porch of our reborn cottage. The entire structure's rotten parts had been demolished, and then it was made whole and sound. I was more than bemused at the irony of how I, too, had been given new life by modern expertise. How fitting that I sat in the same wicker chair on the new porch three years later and reflected about my old and new lives.

My journey had been largely a spiritual and emotional one. Of course the immediate threat of death had taken priority in getting the workups and treatments, but once the medical cards had been played and the course was underway, the challenge was to follow through and stay on top of it all. I knew that the options were to descend into demoralization and self-destruction and, worse, death or to take it on. It boiled down to such a fundamental question. From day one, the overall personal impact of the cancer had been up to me: Was it to be a curse or a gift? Either way, it had been a colossal pain in the ass.

There were few to no remedies for the soaring side effects of prostate inflammation and upside-down hormones. I was physically and emotionally challenged every day and night, especially for the first year and a half, and the looming image of killer cancer didn't help any. Nonetheless, I had to keep my morale strong throughout, that is, I had to hold fast to my purpose and meaning of life. And then there had been the bleeding crisis and the specter of recurrence.

The Reaper must have grinned as I cringed in terror until the question of active cancer was answered at the three-year mark.

I was told after the fact that I'd contended with more fallout than most men. Three years later, all the irritant and obstructive symptoms have gone, and the residual effects from the testosterone shutdown nearly so.

Besides—are you ready for this trite pun?—the alternative would have been deadly.

Speaking of corny expressions, it has been hard to articulate the personal growth from all of this without sounding platitudinous. Many famous historical characters and celebrities have written testimonials and biographies about "rising above a bad situation and making the best of it." There have been plenty of clichés as well as genuinely heart-warming life stories of triumph; I've personally witnessed many thousands in my patients. But my life has been real, my journey has been anything but trite, and my lessons have not been completed. I've learned every inch along the way and continue to do so. Of that much I have been grateful and proud.

Therefore, the shifts and deepening in me were forged in the fire itself. I've noted them along the way, and I included my faltering, just as I had promised that day leaving the hospital in December 2003. The Great Mystery, the Serenity Prayer, the Rule of Holes, and Sutton's Law feel very much a part of who I am now. Add the power of love and faith…and laughs.

So I would have to go with gift, not curse. As a man and as a physician, I'm a bit wiser and certainly more humble than before. I've been forced to face the dark night of seemingly unfathomable injustice, unpredictability, and impotence, just as have many millions of fellow humans. No crisis before had me as painfully aware of how much, and how little, I could do for myself and others.

At first I thought there was nothing I could do to make any difference. The die had been cast, I had cancer, and my fate was in God's hands, prayer or no prayer. But on the beach that first day, I began the process of reconciliation, acknowledging my life landscape and then finding the goods to do my very best every day. Those qualities included faith, love, courage, and persistence—and never forget humor. I took those ideas for granted before, even though I'd earnestly taught them. But for the past three years, they've been living concepts.

******

Several days later I again sat in the wicker chair on the porch, watching the rising sun and hearing the emerging chirping of birds awakening to the morning. Their activity became cheerier as they talked among themselves, probably looking for a breakfast worm or some other bird morsel. Traffic sounds began in the distance, signaling the opening of another day of commerce and travel, and a neighbor's car tires crunched the pebbles in the lane in front of the cottage as he left for the day's adventure.

Rather than feeling smug about my victory, I felt humbled. Yes, modern medicine and my follow-through indeed may have beaten the cancer, at least for now and hopefully for good, but something would kill me sooner or later. So the real victory was in living daily as fully as I could, finding sense in the nonsense, and feeling power in the impotence of life. It had become clear to me that my contending with possible death had been a window into dealing with living. It wasn't over at all; in fact, I would always be challenged to make the most of every day, every moment, right up to my last. There's no place to hide from life's unpredictable fragility.

To this day, I don't know if Susan really had as little fear and apprehension as she portrayed despite our talking about her side of the picture. We certainly talked, and she did admit to the fears and doubts that I'd assumed she had, though in her characteristically understated way. She's deeply intuitive and accepting of life's big picture. I don't mean she's fatalistic because her values are passionately held. Living, not surviving, is as important to her as it is to me.

Anyhow, I still hope she didn't suffer in silence to spare me. Oh, she griped in the second year about the loss of hiking, tennis, and traveling. At first she did the activities on her own, with or without friends; then, as I was able to come back on board, we resumed most aspects of our lives, often with her prodding. So all I can do is take her word for it and observe that she was her usual self throughout the past three years.

As for family and friends, they no longer inquire about how my cancer is or how I'm doing. Once the three-year tests were fine, the issue naturally dropped from conversation, which has been a good thing. I don't feel or act ill, so they must assume that life has returned to normal—and indeed it has in most respects. What lessons any of them might have taken from observing me is only my guess. Early on, I talked with each of the four kids and several friends about experiencing the uncontrollability of life, about taking nothing for granted, and so forth. But now, thankfully, no one sees me as ill or even inconvenienced, and I don't either. I'm just a bit more alive.

******

An afternoon on the porch and I'm alone with my thoughts.

The fire's out and no hot coals appear to be smoldering.

I'm closer than ever to Susan. I cherish my friends more and try not to take life for granted. I find new wisdom in my grandmother's admonition offered every time she heard me complain of a rainy day indoors: "Don't wish your life away, young man."

In fact, I no longer wear a watch after office hours. How could exact punctuality be relevant when hanging out with Susan or friends? How could structured time possibly serve my leisure sports, reading, or meditation? Besides, the gesture of setting aside my weekday timepiece serves as a signal to "chill"—I want to savor each morsel for as long as the flavor lasts. Being in the "now" has new meaning.

And wonder of all wonders, I have several doctors whom I see for both needed treatment and routine monitoring. I have a dentist, dental hygienist, ophthalmologist, urologist, radiation-oncologist, podiatrist, orthopedist, dermatologist, dermatologic surgeon, cardiologist, gastroenterologist, and internist. And I see a massage therapist and energy healer from time to time. Before this sea change, I just went to the dentist and wore glasses updated with a new prescription when my visual acuity decreased. The new lineup partly reflects the march of aging and partly reflects the dissolution of my myth of a being unto myself.

I relish moments of relaxation, and I wouldn't miss a grounding meditation. I cherish my time with Susan, family, and friends. My grandchildren now number seven, and I look forward to being part of their future. Our being in Rhode Island a lot of the time will increasingly remove the geographic barriers to being involved in the daily lives of my extended family. Let's hope we take the chance to make up for lost time.

My admiration for patients' triumphs grows every day. I'm often in awe at the way they are carrying on their lives in the face of grinding heartaches.

******

I rose from the chair, stretched out fully, and took a loving look at the backyard and woods filled with sights and sounds of the waning day. Birds were especially busy wrapping up before dark. Before turning to go inside, I paused with a final thought:

Every six months from now on, I must interrupt the music with a PSA to see if the Reaper is coming to change the score.

And whether shit is happening or not, I'll continue to laughingly tease and joke every chance I get.

*****

Suggested Reading

Benson, Herbert, *Timeless Healing : The Power and Biology of Belief*, Scribner, New York 1996.

Relaxation Response, William Morrow & Co., New York, 1975.

The Mind/Body Effect, Berkley Publishing Group, New York, 1980.

Beyond The Relaxation Response: How to Harness the Healing Power of Your Personal Beliefs, Times Books, New York, 1984.

Your Maximum Mind, Random House, New York, 1987.

Blood, Casey. *Science, Sense and Soul: The Mystical-Physical Nature of Human Existence.* Renaissance Books, 2001

Borysenko, Joan. *Pocketful of Miracles.* Warner Books, 1994

Minding the Body, Mending the Mind. Bantam Books, 1987

Brown, Timothy. *Psalms and Compassions* Resonant Publishing, 2004

Cohen, Richard M. *Blindsided* Harper Collins, 2004

Dossey, Larry: *The Extraordinary Healing Power of Ordinary Things*. Crown Pub. 2006
Reinventing Medicine: Beyond Mind-Body to a New Era of Healing Harper Collins, 1999
Healing Words. The Power of Prayer and the Practice of Medicine. Harper Collins, 1997
Prayer is Good Medicine. Harper Collins, 1996

Dowling Singh, Kathleen. *The Grace in Dying: A Message of Hope, Comfort, and Spiritual Transformation*. Harper San Francisco, 1998

Gerber, Richard. *Vibrational Medicine: The #1 Handbook of Subtle Energy Therapies*. Inner Traditions International, Ltd., 2001

Granet, Roger. *Surviving Cancer Emotionally* John Wiley & Sons, 2001

Gray, Ross. *Prostate Tales: Men's Experiences with Prostate Cancer* Harriman, Tennessee, Men's Studies, 2003

Hapur, Tom. *Finding the Still Point*. Northstone Pub. 2002

Harrington, Anne, editor, *The Placebo Effect: An Interdisciplinary Exploration*, Harvard University Press, Cambridge, 1999.

Holland, Jimmie C. *The Human Side of Cancer: Living with Hope, Coping with Uncertainty,* Memorial Sloan-Kettering Cancer Center, 1999

Jelsing, Nadine. *Prostate Cancer: Portraits of Empowerment,* Westview Press, 1999

Kabat-Zinn, Jon *Full Catastrophe Living, How to Cope with Stress, Pain and Illness Using Mindfulness Meditation,* Judy Piatkus Publishers Ltd London, UK, 1989.

Koenig, Harold G., *Spirituality in Patient Care: Why, How, When, and What*, Templeton Foundation Press, West Conshohocken, Pennsylvania 2002

Korda, Michael. *Man to Man: Surviving Prostate Cancer*, Success Research Corporation, 1997

Lawlis, G, Frank, *Transpersonal Medicine*, Shambhala, Halifax, 1996.

Payne, James E. *Me Too: A Doctor Survives Prostate Cancer*. WRS Publishing

Remen, Naomi. *Kitchen Table Wisdom: Stories That Heal*. Penguin Group, 1996
My Grandfather's Blessings: Stories of Strength, Refuge, and Belonging. Penguin Group, 2001
Mystery: The Wisdom of the Soul. Hay House, 2001

Strobel, Lee, *The Case for Faith : A Journalist Investigates the Toughest Objections to Christianity*. Zondervan Books, Grand Rapids, Michigan, U.S.A, 2000.

Strumolo, Vincent. *"A Fight for Life: Beating Cancer"* Writers Club Press, 2001

Targ, Russell, and Katra, Jane, *Miracles of the Mind: Exploring Nonlocal Consciousness and Spiritual Healing*, New World Library, New York, 1999.

Education, Distinctions, and Experience

Robert J. Mignone, M.D., F.A.P.A.

Education: Amherst College (B.A., Cum Laude), Duke (M.D., B.M.Sc., A.O.A.), Yale (Internal Medicine), Cornell–New York Hospital (Neurology), National Institutes of Health (Neurology), Harvard Medical School, Mass General Hospital (Psychiatry, Chief Resident, Acute Psychiatric Service)

Teaching: Harvard Medical School clinical faculty 1974-1988 University of South Florida Medical and Nursing Schools clinical faculty, University of South Florida undergraduate adjunct faculty (various courses)

Clinical Experience: Founded and worked with Boston North Shore Associates (multi-specialty mental health group in Salem, Massachusetts, and Mass General Hospital) for fifteen years; founded and worked with Gulf Coast Health Services (multi-specialty mental health group with holistic orientation in Sarasota and Venice, Florida, with all ages and modalities represented;

243

gulfcoasthealthservices.com), the largest such group in southwest Florida, for last sixteen years

Certifications and Distinctions: Board Certified, American Board of Psychiatry and Neurology; Fellow, American Psychiatric Association (F.A.P.A.); ordained, Universal Church of the Master; *Sarasota Magazine,* June issue cover story , 2004, 2005, 2006, and 2007 "Top Docs"; voted "Top Psychiatrist in Southwest Florida" by peers in medicine and nursing, based on curriculum vitae and referral prominence--all three years of its running. Numerous regional teaching sessions and workshops as well as many television appearances and radio shows

Marketing: Gifted public speaker and media talent who welcomes challenge.

About the Author

Robert J. Mignone, M.D., F.A.P.A.

Dr. Mignone's thirty five years of full time clinical practice have enriched his cumulative admiration for the courage of the many thousands of alarmed and shocked souls he has attended in their attempts to bounce back from all manner of crises. Cancer has been just one. This time it was his turn to face the dark night and find the meaning and purpose to go on. His journey was maturing, to say the least—so, being the teacher that he has always been—he now offers his memoir for learning.

As his practice has grown in Southwest Florida he has taught, lectured, written, and used media to reach out to the community. He has been called a gifted and inspirational speaker—in person and on TV. From 2004 to 2007 the *Sarasota Magazine* has run a cover feature on Top Docs in each specialty in Southwest Florida. The designations derived from peer votes and recommendations/nominations, curriculum vitae, teaching and clinical experience. The Castle Connoly Research Group and *Sarasota Magazine* have cited Mignone as Top Psychiatrist for all four years of the feature publication.

His upcoming book, *Psychiatric Injury: Evaluation and Treatment of Psychiatric Impairment,* reflects a different side of Dr. Mignone. It is less a memoir—more a practical handbook—for judges, lawyers, insurance professionals, and physicians involved with the field of disability medicine, especially Workers Compensation. He offers the Medical Model of anti-regressive and sound scholarship of contemporary psychiatry as a balance between the poles of adversarial argument. Psychiatry's credibility in this niche gets a solid boost. For twenty plus years he has participated in trial and deposition proceedings, has consulted to attorneys and insurance professionals, and has examined thousands of injured and disabled men and women. This handbook reflects that accumulated experience.

Printed in the United States
107687LV00002B/1-30/A

9 781598 009309